06 - 29 - 15

To D Bradley Taylor

Do good, not to show others
good in return,
but it is right to do

Sincerely

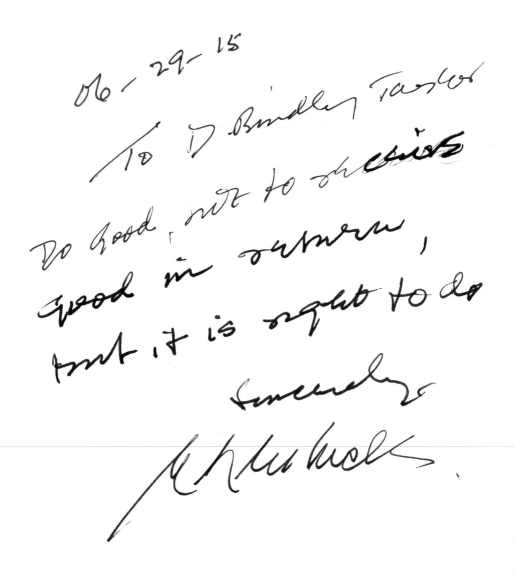

THE HEALTH
CARE DILEMMA

THE HEALTH CARE DILEMMA

An Inside View

Randolph R. Estwick, MSc., MD., FACP

Xlibris LLC
1-888-795-4274
www.Xlibris.com
602564

CONTENTS

To those players in health care who have given
much but received little in return

ACKNOWLEDGMENT

I am appreciative and grateful to my wife, Kay, without whose dedication, support, and encouragement this book would not have been possible. Even during her illness, when strength in her left upper extremity had diminished and walking became difficult, her critique remained undisputable. She would find a period or a quotation omitted, comma inappropriately placed, or a word incorrectly spelled. I was always reluctant to have her read a chapter which had already been posted; she would invariably find a valid error.

Her illness and her succeeding hospitalization have given me depth and insight to some of the problems and the dilemma in the delivery of health care which many citizens experience and accept as a way of life. Her moral support and her intellectual contributions have given me the strength to endure and overcome periods of frustration and uncertainty in the completion of this book during the final days. It is largely through her input that I am able to share the thoughts and frustrations of many senior citizens with similar experience.

I acknowledge those physicians and health workers who dedicate their lives to caring for the elderly and the disabled, even refusing more lucrative pursuits. I also extend my appreciation to Dr. Louise Dunbar Robbins for her timely review of the manuscript before it was finally reviewed by the publishers. Much appreciation is extended to *The New York Times* for their excellent reporting of health care issues and events, bringing to focus issues which may otherwise be buried under the guise of correctness.

Finally, I acknowledge with appreciation insurance representatives, administrators, nurses, social workers, care workers, and patients who were very receptive and generous in their time and their answers to many searching questions; their contributions added credence to many of the events and the information referenced in this book.

PRELUDE

I have given an inside view of my perception of the heath care dilemma. I was motivated by my daily experience with my wife who has suffered from the sudden onset of a stroke. This experience has brought me face-to-face with occurrences and situations which were alien to me as a physician and consultant in physical medicine and rehabilitation. Many events included here were previously disclosed by the press or published by government or private agencies. Some of this information may have escaped the attention of readers. Interpretation and presentation of events, however, are based on experience gained by years of practice in the field of medicine; this is in contrast to the experience of a layman whose spouse has suffered a major medical event. I found myself in the very unique position of being "two persons in one," the experienced physician on one side of the coin and the spouse of the victim of a major medical event—a stroke—on the other side. My task as an author is to present perspectives which I could not envisage as a physician. I have concluded that it was easier as a physician. Many of the events encountered were unthinkable and unknown to the author.

I have now brought into focus two sides of the same coin. The view from inside has revealed that there are many players in the field of health care delivery, all of whom exert some influence in its delivery. What is disconcerting is the fact that none of the players has taken any responsibility for its unbridled and escalating cost; they all believe that it is the responsibility of the other player. Therefore, nothing is done to reduce the cost of health care and the unconscionable burden on Middle America. I have mentioned important players in the field who may be contributors to this dilemma and have cited some of their contributions. The intent here is to be more informative. Ideas presented are not intended as gospel but merely another point of view. Readers may expand their thoughts by reading original manuscripts and reports available for public scrutiny.

Senior care, skilled nursing facilities, independent living facilities, and the role of physical medicine and rehabilitation are all discussed at some length. Issues and concerns obliquely related to health care were also discussed; these include long-term insurance coverage, the immigrants' contributions to health care, and the most precious years of our lives, "the golden years." Finally, an overview of the dilemma in health care was given in the context of a physician.

PROLOGUE

This book is not intended as a critique of the health care system. Many of the players, physicians and care workers who maintain the system, are caring and dedicated. Physicians, with whom I have spoken, have elected to labor in the system, foregoing more lucrative opportunities elsewhere; they deserve our appreciation and plaudits. It is not the intent to offer remedies, although this may be perceived in some instances. I have attempted to expose some of the realities encountered in my travail through a system which is as sick as the clients/*patients* under its care. It is my hope that others may propose and effect solutions. *The Health Care Dilemma: An Inside View* emanated from my personal experience after a close family member required hospitalization, subacute rehabilitation, home care, and skilled nursing care (SNC), following a stroke (cerebrovascular accident [CVA]). I have had to navigate through a maze of bureaucrats, functionaries, and the folks whom I have come to regard as the real pillars of the system, the health care workers, the caregivers.

As a physician who spent virtually all of his professional years as a specialist in physical medicine and rehabilitation, my experience is unique, although not fully appreciated nor recognized by those whose perspicacity is clouded by other issues. For the purpose of this book, I am no longer the chief of service and director of a department at a county hospital. I suddenly became a rank-and-file layman whose loved one had suffered an unexpected life-threatening event. My emotion was heightened; my thinking and my ability to make an objective assessment at that moment were blunted. I felt then that it was easier to function as a chief of service or a medical director than as the spouse of a victim of this unexpected event, a stroke. Formulating a treatment plan and writing a definitive prescription for my patients were all relatively easier to undertake as a physician, but I am no longer a physician.

I suddenly realized that my perception of these events as an attending physician and as they affected patients and their loved ones was erroneous. I am now convinced that only the victims and their loved ones can fully grasp the full dimension and ramifications of these illnesses when they occur within a family. The coin looks very differently on the other side, the patient's side, the family side. I have since developed more humility, more compassion, more empathy, and more contrition now than as an attending physician. The question then becomes, can a physician fully appreciate the anguish and suffering experienced by his patients and their loved ones during these critical events? My answer is unequivocally no. To fully appreciate, one must experience; if this were not so, those who race automobiles at 240 miles per hour and those who pursue the most dangerous and daring sports "just for the satisfaction" would be quite content to read about these events or see them performed. However, they chose to experience the events by performing them. It is hoped that my disclosure will serve to improve the care of those who are physically challenged, especially the stroke victim.

Recent press report about a white South African family was quite telling: The family had a living experience they may never forget: the gated community versus the Phomolong squatter camp, Mamelodi South Africa. Here is the story of a white South African family who had been accustomed to the aplomb of white middle-class South African lifestyle in a country which had rigidly maintained the most repressive apartheid regime against native black South Africans.

The family lived in absolute comfort and luxury in a gated Pretoria estate home but decided to experience life in its fullness and majesty in a depressed and degraded African community. This meant that the family of four, two adults and two children, would be living in a one-hundred-square-foot shack for one month, the month believed to be one of the bleakest months of the year under conditions which millions of black South Africans have endured as a way of life for years. The family took with them nothing that may enhance their quality of life and comfort. There was no running water; the outdoor pit latrine was shared with neighbors; they depended on public transportation just like others in the community. No one but this family can fully appreciate the full impact of this self-imposed austere living, whatever the motives or objectives may have been. Reading about the most complicated surgical procedures and observing them being performed by the most proficient surgeon are not sufficient for acquisition of the skills necessary to be a good practitioner. The very term medical practitioner implies practice, i.e., "to perform repeatedly," not merely to read or to observe. To grasp the innate experience of victims and loved ones, the doctor must shed the "umbrella of the white coat and stethoscope" and live on the other side of the coin, the patient's side.

I am certain that no textbook reports, no documentary, or the most evocative presentation by news reporters could have given this South African family the knowledge they received by living in that community. It is one thing to read about outdoor "pit latrines." It is quite different to use one located at some distance from your sleeping quarters, doors without locks, accumulated waste in a pit cleared once or twice a year, where discarded newspaper, in lieu of toilet paper, is seen as a luxury and washing of the hands an extravagance; slots designed for ventilation are wide enough to facilitate free entry of snakes and curious eyes. You would only fully appreciate the onerous effects of these conditions if you have lived them. I believe there is integration of many intangible forces operating in the minds of those who are implicated, which no one else can fully appreciate, including physicians or care workers.

I woke up about seven thirty that memorable morning, March 20, 2012. My wife was already awake and informing me about the weather forecast for the day, not realizing what had occurred to her during the night. During her preoccupation about the weather, predicted to be scattered sunshine, I was reflecting on my sojourn as a medical student in the United Kingdom. Whenever one saw a glimmer of sunshine early in the day, it was a common morning salutation to say "It's a rather nice day, isn't it?" It did not matter how foreboding the rest of the sky appeared. When I turned around and looked at Kay's left arm then lifted it, it was flaccid (lifeless). I immediately said to her, "Kay, I think you had a stroke during the night."

She replied as clearly as ever, "You got to be kidding."

The impact on me and the ramifications did not penetrate until sometime later. I then examined her more carefully to confirm my initial impression. She had in fact suffered a stroke, a right CVA with left upper weakness. She is right-handed, so I reasoned that with a left paresis, her speech may be spared, my reasoning being that her speech component would more likely be in her left cerebral area. Whether my reasoning was correct or not is now irrelevant; her speech was intact. Having managed stroke patients for a number of years, I was convinced this was a stroke in evolution, and the sooner we got to the emergency room, the better.

"STROKE IN EVOLUTION" brought back to memory a telephone call I received from the press. Tuesday, April 19, 1994, I had just arrived at my office when my secretary called me to say "A reporter from the press." It transpired that a former president of the United States had been stricken by a stroke on Monday, April 18, 1994, and he had been taken to a New York hospital. He was being treated in the intensive care unit. The reporter said, "I am phoning you because I learned that you have considerable rehabilitation experience with victims of stroke as a rehabilitation specialist and a consultant at the local hospital." I was flattered that the press would seek my opinion on the prognosis of a critical medical event affecting a former president of the United States. However, I reasoned that I was not dealing with a president of the United States; I was dealing with a human person, a stroke victim. I had been in the practice of physical medicine and rehabilitation for many years and managed a number of stroke patients. I was fully credentialed and certified, even served as an expert witness in court. I was up to the task. There was no difference in my competence as a specialist in physical medicine and rehabilitation than that of the consultant in internal medicine at the center where the former president was being treated.

According to the press release, the president's physician was reported to have said, "The former president will be moved out of intensive care to a private room later on Tuesday," saying "he was out of danger" and described him as "awake, alert and in good spirit, and able to understand." He said, "The former president suffered paralysis on his right side. No dramatic changes are anticipated in his condition over the next several days." The reporter wanted to have my views on the former president's condition and my prognosis. The following is a quote from my interview with the press on that day and was stated in layman's terms:

> "A stroke occurs when a blood vessel carrying oxygen to the brain bursts or is blocked. Physicians generally like to wait twenty-four to forty-eight hours before giving a prognosis on a stroke victim," said Dr. Randolph Estwick, director of physical medicine and rehabilitation at Pascack Valley Hospital in Westwood. "During this period, the condition of the patient is most likely still evolving," said Estwick, who said he did not have all the details of the president's stroke. "After that period, one can make some prediction as to outcome, and even then, you're not sure how much the recovery will be until they get started in rehabilitation."

As it transpired, the former president's condition took turn for the worse, and he expired several days later. It was clear that this was only a press interview, and I had no part in the actual treatment of the former president. Nevertheless, I received several phone calls from would-be patients from as far as Pennsylvania who had read the article and wanted to make appointments—fame by osmosis.

My wife insisted that she did not wish to be transported by an ambulance, with all the commotion this would entail at eight o'clock in the morning, especially in an environment where most residents seem to enjoy their morning snooze and luxuriate in their retirement. There was little time to convince her otherwise. I donned her robe and was able to get her in my car. Within fifteen to twenty minutes, we were at the hospital emergency room. Since the onset of her stroke was probably well over three hours ago, it was not considered appropriate to administer the tissue plasminogen activator (T-PA) at the emergency room. TPA is usually administered intravenously. It is a thrombolytic agent for ischemic stroke given within three hours of the onset of an ischemic event. When the term *ischemic stroke* is used, it generally implies a stroke which is not caused by a bleeding episode, within or directly outside of the brain, which is described as a cerebral hemorrhage.

Waiting in the ER seemed endless. There were long periods when nothing seemed to have taken place. The emphasis was on details about our insurance coverage. Now I am not a consultant. I am not a physician. I am just the ordinary Joe sweating it out in the emergency room of a hospital and anxiously pacing the floor. I murmured to myself, "When in hell are they going to see my wife?" The other faculty in me said, "Calm down, Randy. Your wife is not in pain. She did not have a heart attack or a cerebral hemorrhage." I then fully understood the anguish and anxiety experienced by thousands of family members and patients who enter emergency rooms throughout the country. For most of these people, a reassuring word would go a long way to soothe their souls and calm their anxieties. Very often, such solace is missing. It seldom comes from the top of the totem pole, the physician. On that memorable day, my hero was the emergency room nurse; she was reassuring and informed me that the attending physician was notified and what they planned to accomplish before the doctor arrives. She offered me a seat next to my wife; she offered me coffee or tea. There was a reassuring demeanor in everything she did. The ER doctor arrived later; he introduced himself and gave me a briefing about his findings and his plans, pending consultation with her physician. He was quite detached but professional and respectful. The ER nurse managed to inject a soft smile when she spoke to me in spite of the many procedures she carried out. The doctor was somber, perhaps a replica of myself as an emergency room physician, the other side of the coin.

I was reminded of the experience of a friend who was an attending urologist and chief of service at a large teaching university hospital in Michigan. He became seriously ill and was admitted as a patient to the same hospital. He spent over four weeks in the intensive care unit and the urological service.

"I saw the medical students, the residents, consultant urologists, professor, and chair of the Department of Urology. They appeared in their white coats almost every day, some with stethoscopes dangling from their ears. They all seemed so intimidating, I felt worse every time they came around my bed," he told me he was near death. After his recovery and was discharged from hospital, he began writing a book. One of the questions he asked in his book was: "Who was the most important person in restoring my health?" Before he volunteered the answer, I felt surely it was his chief resident. They are usually "the chief cook and bottle washer," to quote an old saying. To my surprise, this distinguished physician mentioned in his book the name of the woman who cleaned his room every day she was on duty. He stated:

> The medical team was good in the service they rendered, but during their ward rounds, they all spoke over me and among themselves. I often felt death was imminent by the whispers I could not hear nor understand and the absence of their eye contact. No one seemed to look at me.
>
> The cleaning woman, whom I had upstaged to "the cleaning lady," spoke directly to me and to my fears. She was always reassuring as she mopped under and around my hospital bed. Before leaving my private room, which incidentally only imposed another level of unnecessary isolation, she would always touch me gently and say to me: "Doc, you gonna be *ah right*." Those last words were powerful and therapeutic; they meant more to me at that time than the clinical examination skillfully performed by the resident physician.

The emergency rooms at many hospitals need more personnel like the cleaning lady at this Michigan hospital. The hiatus in the E.R. was followed by the usual clinical work up. Eventually, the neurologist arrived to give her pronouncement, which was already known, and my wife was admitted to the subacute intensive care unit. By the time I left the hospital, the weakness in her left lower extremity, which was only minimally affected when we left home, had become more severe in keeping with the process of an evolving stroke. After three days at the acute care hospital, she was transferred to a subacute physical rehabilitation facility where her definitive rehabilitation program began.

I was quite composed, so I thought, through all the stresses and strains related to my wife's sudden illness and her subsequent admission to hospital. I did not realize nor did I fully appreciate how much this experience had impacted my emotion until I got home that evening and tried to sleep. My eyes would close, the external ocular muscles were too fatigued to keep them open, but my mind was well awake. It was very difficult to reconcile the thought that my wife may not be able to function as she did prior to this event. In my work as a specialist in physical medicine and rehabilitation (PM&R), it was relatively easy to prognosticate. I had done this before as an expert witness. Now I can hardly find words to make a relatively easy diagnosis, much more a prognosis. There was too much denial in processing the information I was receiving from the various clinical sources, though in the past, I had no problem doing this as a specialist.

The entire encounter left me wiser but humbler, not wisdom in the academic sense but in the vulnerability of man. It *made me more cognizant of my humanity and frailties* after I had cast aside the doctor's comport.

STATISTICS ON STROKE

An overview of the stroke syndrome: It is believed that between five hundred thousand and six hundred thousand people living in the United States will suffer from the effects of a stroke. Of this number, about one hundred thousand or more may die as a result. About two hundred fifty thousand find their way to rehabilitation centers. Stroke ranks about third as a cause of death in the United States. It is also one of the main causes of long-term illness and disability. It is a misconception to believe that this syndrome is peculiar only to the aged; young people also suffer this tragic illness.

It is not the intent of this publication to detail the treatment of acute or long-term stroke. I have shared my experience with a stroke victim, not to be confused with a victim of central cervical cord compression syndrome, which may also result in paralysis and about which I have previously published in some detail in *Geriatrics*. Suffice to alert readers of the risk factors, many of which are treatable. I have always concurred with the view that the best way to treat a stroke patient is to prevent it from occurring. Treat aggressively those treatable risk factors. Simply put, risk factors are those conditions and/or indulgences which, when many occur in one's medical history or practiced extensively, may result in a stroke.

SOME ESTABLISHED RISK FACTORS:

- Hypertension/preexisting heart disease and atrial fibrillation
- Diabetes
- *Tobacco smoking*
- Excessive alcohol consumption

*This vice not only reduces oxygen in the blood, but it also influences narrowing of the arteries. My grandmother was more explicit in describing the act of smoking as "fire at one end and a damn fool at the other end." This simplistic view is not shared by the author; the habit is pernicious. One of my patients, who always suffered chest pain after smoking, would plea for a "pain medicine" rather than giving up the cigarette. I would always assure him that he has the lever that triggers his chest pain and he should use it wisely. He was still smoking when I left that service.

- Obesity
- A previous stroke or TIA (transient ischemic attack)
- High blood cholesterol
- A sedentary lifestyle
- **Ethnicity/Heredity*
- Sex; men are at higher risk and at younger age
- Aging; longer life, greater probability
- Atherosclerosis
- Some oral contraceptives and illegal intravenous drug use

**African Americans and Hispanics are said to have a higher risk of disability from a stroke.

Many risk factors (hypertension/atrial fibrillation, high blood cholesterol, diabetes, and obesity) are generally treatable by your local MD and/or in consultation with a specialist/internist. The indulgences (cigarette smoking, illegal IV drug use) are in your hands. Do something about them.

This introduction is a prelude to evolution of the health care dilemma. Stroke patients are more likely to be relegated to the status of chronic illness with all its appendages. Many of these patients have used up their Medicare benefits and without coverage for skilled nursing care. Home care and conversion of their status to Medicaid may be the only alternative for these victims. Those who are fortunate to have some long-term care (LTC) insurance coverage may find that to initiate these benefits by your insurance carriers is sometimes like extracting an intransigent molar tooth by an inexperienced dental practitioner.

The skillful and experienced social worker may be able to convert the status of some of these elder citizens so that alternative and often obscured benefits may become available. I have high regard for social workers who are often some of the most dedicated personnel in the chain of command. They fight an uphill battle with insurance carriers, hospital administrators, physicians, even with relatives and the victims themselves. In the end, I have to salute them because they eventually get the job done and able to extract a smile from all the stakeholders.

We are still faced with a sick and disabled human being whose basic needs require partial or full assistance of the human hands to provide for his/her daily needs. These individuals are prime candidates for other institutional care (nursing home, long-term care, assisted care). Alternatively, they may be transferred from the acute care hospital to their respective homes where they receive home care. For many, such alternative may be their greatest dilemma—no homes to live and no insurance coverage for their care. Once the determination is made, those with homes and some financial independence may elect to remain in their homes with some assistance and/or supervision by a caregiver or home aide. Others with little or no finances may inevitably end in a chronic or long-term care facility covered by Medicaid insurance. In any event, a home care worker is needed, many of whom are required to give total care to their clients. Such questions often arise: Who are the stakeholders? Who are these workers? I have interviewed a number of them and visited a number of institutions to give you a glimpse of the places and the people you have entrusted to care for your loved ones and the dilemma encountered.

I would be remiss if I failed to mention the extraordinary cost in the delivery of health care in the United States. Many years ago, this was a popular expression: "Don't get sick overseas, especially in a developing country." Today some use the same expression with a different reference: "Don't get sick in the United States." We now see an increasing number of Americans traveling to the far corners of the world to receive comparable health care at a cost they can afford.

HEALTH CARE DELIVERY in the United States is now largely relegated to profit making, sometimes at any cost irrespective of claims to the contrary. The increasing number of health-related facilities springing up throughout the country, the untenable rates they charge for their occupancy and care, the executives and boards which control and dictate their policies are testaments to their penchant for profit making. There is little I have experienced, *viewing from inside*, to convince me that the operation of these institutions has any primary interest in the benevolence of the clients they serve and the society at large. One institution has had the temerity to announce in advance of occupancy that they will institute extra charges for the very diaper worn by seniors or those clients who must use them; they have finally reached the lowest ebb in institutional charges. This is the extent to which the "playing field" has now degenerated in order to extract another dollar from some coerced, entrapped, and hapless victims.

Any attempt to resolve the escalating cost in the health care madness must first identify the contributors in order of culpability then there must be an admission of guilt. I have reasons to report that victims, the insured, also share a measure of guilt, so no one is exempt. Other facilities have charged for items which were already provided by clients/patients.

The pharmaceutical conglomerates

The insurance conglomerates

The health care conglomerates and their operating executives

The physicians—and non-physicians-operated medical/surgical groups

The inadvertent patients

The Players
And Attitudes

Who are the players in the health care dilemma? They are the countless men and women who toil every day to care for the sick and disabled. Many of these workers are subjected to humiliation and perhaps work at the lowest pay scale of any workforce, yet they carry on to maintain the pyramid described in this book. The players are the senior citizens cared for at their homes or at the various institutions, who, on occasion, bear the brunt of the dishonest and the abusive caregiver. The players are the large institutions and their corporate executives who would spare nothing to enhance their already enhanced salaries and bonuses. Finally, the players are all those who use the system: the pharmaceutical giants, the insurance conglomerates, the physicians, and their patients.

Players in the health care debacle include the health care agencies which provide personnel and/or equipment, the physicians, the institutions (nursing homes, skilled nursing facilities (SNF), acute care hospitals, and rehabilitation centers), the caregivers (aides), and the clients/patients and family members who have the on-going responsibility for overseeing the health care management of their loved ones. Peripherally, mention should be made of long-term insurance (LTI) carriers. Regretfully, some of these institutions procrastinate in fulfillment of their fiduciary obligations and impose every roadblocks to their transparency.

Most health care agencies are for-profit organizations established for the purpose of providing personnel who care for or offer therapy to the sick and disabled who otherwise may be unable to avail themselves with the skilled professionals they need. Some agencies only provide health-care-related equipment for purchase or rental, such as wheelchairs, orthotic (splints and braces) or prosthetic (artificial limbs) devices; most accept Medicare/Medicaid reimbursements for equipment prescribed by physicians. Important participants are agencies which provide personnel, including the aides. These agencies are providing professional services, serving physicians, registered nurses, licensed practical nurses, physical and occupational therapists, and speech therapists. The core of my experience relates to the aides, the people who provide hands-on day-to-day care for your loved ones. Who are these people? You may be enlightened to get a glimpse of these caregivers, the base of the health care pyramid, many of whom are hardworking, caring and dedicated human beings. Yet many of them endure insults and humiliation from their very dependent clients and/or their family members. Not uncommonly, these servants react in ways which are perceived as cruel and inhuman; in fact, they very well may be.

Interviewing those who work as independent contractors and those working through health care agencies revealed work experiences which were shocking and troublesome, ranging from very low pay ($8 an hour) to poor and demeaning treatment of the aide workers. Independent contractors negotiate their wages directly with their clients/patients or family members and are paid directly by their clients. Their wages are significantly higher, and for the most part, they receive no other benefits; most home care workers prefer this arrangement. They negotiate their own contract for wages and insurance payments. They receive more cash in hand and are able to make independent decisions about their financial affairs.

What is it like to work as a home care aide/caregiver? My inquiry was revealing.

ATTITUDES: Most of the workers interviewed were people of color, with the exception of a nursing director and a nurse consultant. The claim of racial undertones was not uncommon, and in many instances, the perpetrators were oblivious of this malady. The debased attitude of some clients and their family members toward their caregivers was so pervasive that any person of color entering or leaving these institutions was subjected to the same humiliating experience. As medical director of the department of physical medicine and rehabilitation at a county hospital and a consultant at one of the institutions evaluated, I was not exempt from this unsavory and sinister behavior perpetrated against people of color, even those serving the needs of the sick and disabled.

Leaving one health care facility where I was a consultant, I observed an elderly male gentleman with a caregiver pushing his spouse in a standard wheelchair; she was apparently a disabled individual. As the aide struggled pushing her obese client, the exit door was about to close as the chair entered; afraid that the door would slam into her face, I rushed forward and held the closing door to facilitate their safe exit. As the chair exited the door, I was half expecting, at the very least, a "thank you" from the man and certainly from his disabled spouse. Instead, what I received may shock some readers. This woman looked me straight into my eyes and said, "Oh! We can surely use you as our doorman at my apartment building in Hackensack."

I was dumbfounded and could not find words to respond at that moment, and fearful of making an inappropriate remark, I said nothing. My well-pressed suit, stethoscope in my pocket, and, more importantly, my civility in holding the door for the safe exit of a disabled meant nothing to those thankless creatures. Many aides I have interviewed for this publication have expressed similar or worst experiences at the hands of some of the worst elements of our society. To be disrespectful to those who serve the pressing needs of anyone is a dilemma tough to reconcile. My colleague in Psychiatry described this attitude as "Psycho-impediment which may require electro-convulsive therapy (shock therapy) to dislodge." I did not support his assessment as a serious solution.

Regrettably, I have found elements of disrespect live and well today as experienced in the past and referred here in this publication. One's qualifications, expertise, or experience are often obscured by what meets the eye, one's pigmentation. The good news, it is not pervasive. I mention this only to remind readers that "all is not well" and some writers are reluctant to bring their experiences to light and expose them for what they are. My conversations with physicians of color have supported my "inside view." In many cases, the offenders are oblivious of their actions and of the consequences of the thoughts and pronouncements they express; others are deliberate and calculated with the venomous intent to do harm and inflict mental and emotional stress to their targets. These physicians relate experiences where they were relegated in reference to kitchen helpers, aides, and care workers, although their dress, deportment, and work performances were contrary; one does not work in the kitchen with a stethoscope in his pocket, except the chef is expected to have a cardiac arrest. Some physicians are never addressed as physicians as do their professional counterparts, although introduced as physicians; it is as though this denial will relieve them of their knowledge and their standing in the annals of medicine or surgery. In more sophisticated cases, they may be referred to by their surnames, and if they are lucky, the handle "mister" may precede their names. One administrator, I am told, had the temerity to refer to physicians of color by their Christian names, a designation reserved for family, friends, and professional colleagues. This is administrative decorum at its lowest and should be addressed. I suggest that such crude behavior is calculated with an agenda and perpetrated to diminish the standing of the victims, but in fact, it diminishes the standing, if any, of the perpetrators. The fact that the physicians may have had a more rigorous and higher standard of training than the administrator was irrelevant. The thoughts were influenced by a cynical mind with a total disregard for truth and reality; the culture created by such conduct is inimical to quality care.

There is no inherent evil in addressing one by his/her Christian name. The sinister intent enters the equation when this is calculated and selective.

What is not commonly realized and appreciated, such conduct, especially on the part of supervisors and administrators, undermines their authority, diminishes their respect and control; they are viewed as just objects in dark suits whose greatest satisfaction and pleasure come not from work achievement and accomplishments but by giving vent to a suppressed feeling of inadequacy and very low esteem, which the smartest suits will not supplant. Perhaps more importantly, such conduct undermines quality care at these institutions, for most care workers do identify with victims of such crass and unsavory behavior and will react accordingly. A reminder, "respect begets respect." A popular Jamaican expression places everything in context: "It ain't easy, you know!"

During my more thoughtful moments, I asked, from which planet did those beings originate? It is unfortunate and regrettable that people of color seem to be less respected and held in lower esteem, even when they perform tasks and services in the most exemplary manner, some of which are lifesaving. I am certain most of these workers have no desire or inclination to break into any socially restricted society or enter into an alien society; they only wish to be accorded the same human recognition and decency accorded to their white counterparts who perform similar tasks or services—no more, no less. This expectation still eludes many who are the backbones in the care of the nation's sick and disabled.

I have seen evidence of similar behavior perpetrated by those poisoned by hate, ignorance, and disrespect, even for the president of these United States. These shameless offenders are apparently ignorant of the fact that their disrespect is not of the occupant but upon the office of the president; whoever occupies that coveted office in the future will be diminished by their cavalier actions.

In my book, *A Successful Journey, Not Without Pain*, I shared my experience of similar behavior of some professional colleagues. It was disgusting and painful, but my journey was successful because it transcended the petty behavior of some colleagues and focused on something higher and nobler. The undertone of these savage and hostile behavior seem to have shown little change over decades, yet one must continue to hope, and this must always be kept alive. A verse I came across sometime ago seems appropriate, paraphrased, "Do good not to receive good in return, but it is the right thing to do."

Those who employ home care aides to care for their loved ones may wittingly or unwittingly cast insults and repeat them unaware of the harm they may inflict upon others. Remember, these workers are human beings; they do perform an important service, one which you are unwilling or unable to perform. Respect them for the work they do, if not for their humanity.

I listened to one employer extolling the woman she had contracted to care for her elderly father who was suffering from Alzheimer's dementia. She had nothing but praise for this employee who had worked with the family for over five years, "My girl prepares Dad's meals and eats with him. He makes such a mess when he eats."

In my paranoia, I suspected her plaudit for her helper was empty and too hollow to be accepted. They were patently hypocritical, and I thought if she kept running her mouth long enough, her condescending and racist undertone would soon emerge. I was dead on track.

She continued, "Alice is good with Dad, but I don't trust her with my good china. She already broke two of my best cups."

When I could no longer tolerate some of her diatribes, I interrupted her and asked, "How old a female has to be before you addressed her by her name or as a woman?"

Addressing her sixty-one-year-old female home care helper as "my girl" was more than I could have swallowed. Her helper was deemed to be distrustful not because of any mistreatment of her dad but simply because she had broken two replaceable cups. It was as though the cups were of greater importance in establishing trust than the good care of her dad.

She seemed stunned by my rebuke. "Alice doesn't mind," she said. "I do it all the time. We treat her like a member of the family"—the usual cliché often used by some people who disrespect their most trusted employees, especially those of color.

Alice then smiled broadly. To this, the employer said, "See! She is laughing."

My interpretation of Alice's smile was entirely different. Alice ate with her dad as a loyal and dutiful companion. She was being paid to carry out that task, but the truth was the daughter could not stomach her dad's drooling while she sat and eat with him. In her world, a drooling dad was intolerable to sit with during her meal. Having Alice dine with her dad was not because of her affection for Alice or even respect. It was entirely one of necessity and convenience; Alice knew "she could not stomach her dad's drooling." For her tolerance and loyalty, Alice was unjustly rewarded by being characterized as "my girl Alice" at age sixty-one and a grandmother. The irony, her employer saw nothing wrong with her disparaging and condescending characterization of a loyal helper. In some respect the isolation of her drooling father was like the rejection of the blind from dining in residential dining facilities because they required assistance in feeding; yet children are fed in these facilities. The larger question: Is rejection because of "assisted feeding" or because of "being blind?" There is legal recourse for such blatant discrimination.

Alice may have been showing her teeth, but I assure you that Alice was not laughing. There is a well-known Guyanese saying which accurately characterized Alice's inner feeling which her employer could not perceive: "Every time one shows his/her teeth (grins) does not indicate laughter; the tiger also showed its teeth but was preparing for an onslaught."

Another home care worker told me that she was employed for an 8:00 p.m. to 8:00 a.m. shift by a skilled nursing facility to protect a client/patient who suffered dementia but had many lucid moments. This individual was in the habit of wandering during the night. One evening, the client/patient insisted on getting out of her bed. When the female home care helper attempted to restrain her, she became angry and belligerent. The care helper then withdrew in her attempt to restrain. The client yelled at her, "Take your dirty black hands off me, you b—n—," then spat on her face.

"What did you do?" I asked.

"I reported it to my supervisor."

"What did the supervisor do?"

"She told me don't pay her any attention, she doesn't know what she is doing. She is a bit off tonight."

I asked her, "Did you continue to care for her through the night?"

She answered, "Yes! What can I do? I need my job. I need the money."

It was difficult for me to understand how any human being could be subjected to such indignities yet carry out their duties and unpleasant responsibilities as though they were being treated like celebrities with utmost respect. I believe this issue was handled poorly by the supervisor. It left the caregiver with the erroneous impression that her encounter, to be spat upon, was insignificant and goes with the territory of working as a home care provider. It may also have met the old axiom "The customer/patient is always right." Well, this may "hold water" when you are a customer at one of the elite boutiques in Beverly Hills and paying big bucks for small items. It does not "wash" when one is dependent on the good grace and benevolence of a human person, the health care worker. The human element invariably comes into play, and one's action often evokes a reciprocal reaction. I was impressed by the composure and the forbearance of this caregiver whose reaction could only be described as magnanimous in spite of such despicable behavior; she was in fact the hero in this altercation. I would have treated this matter quite differently. I would have confronted this client in the presence of the caregiver, notwithstanding her dementia. I would have highlighted the compassion, the forbearance, and the generosity of spirit in this caregiver in a way which directly relates to the patient's well-being; I would have contrasted these with the negative and insulting behavior of the patient/client.

What if the caregiver had reciprocated by spitting on the patient's face, "an eye for an eye"? This response I would have considered to be totally unacceptable. I have yet to see a person with dementia walk into a blazing fire; this may be simplistic but may have some relevance for many home care workers faced with such intolerance.

It is tempting to suggest that one's approach to these racial issues reflects a "generic and social upbringing." Mental or physical illnesses merely rekindle latent/dormant capacity to disrespect people whose appearances are different. To state it more crudely, a common expression is paraphrased: "Putting lipstick on a pig will not change its characteristics."

I served as a specialist in physical medicine at a psychiatric facility with a wide range of mental disorders; those patients coming from an orderly and respectful social environment hardly ever used the unprintable profanities or engage in actions which are incendiary, even under extreme provocation. My observation has been too consistent to be regarded merely as an incident, although one must keep in mind the rare exception.

Caregivers are not beyond the capacity for hostile conduct toward their charges. It is sad to report that ill-temper and sometimes hostile attitudes are meted out to the disabled and cause greater harm than those experienced by any caregiver. It should not be forgotten that those confined to skilled nursing care, for the most part, are very dependent; they are more vulnerable since many are physically and/or mentally challenged. They have virtually no defense against the vicious actions or omissions of the unscrupulous caregivers and, at worse, may have to endure the neglect imposed by these workers for extended periods. To be confined, to be dependent, then to be abused in any form is inimical to the health and well-being of anyone. Conversely, caregivers have the freedom to go and come as they desire—to work or not to work. Most skilled nursing residents do not enjoy these luxuries. They are told what to eat, when to eat, when to shower, when to retire to bed, what programs to view or to hear. These impositions and deprivations, especially when cognition is intact, are intolerable. There must be a way to relieve the pain, anguish, and frustrations of individuals so structured and restricted. Many of the unwanted behavior and reactions of clients/patients are the only outlets to express their pent-up unhappiness and frustrations.

The health care workers must have the capacity for tolerance and the ability to appreciate the burden imposed by confinement, even in the best SNF. There could be no greater dehumanizing experience than having a lone male caregiver, a total stranger, attending the personal hygiene care of a female senior citizen who was erroneously presumed not to have understood what was going on.

These and other "inside views" must be exposed to evoke better and more considerate care for all those confined to these facilities. The very supervisors who impose and condone these practices would not subject themselves to these practices under similar circumstances. They will not practice what they preach. Few physicians would dare do a GYN exam in the absence of a female attendant.

The knee-jerk reaction of supervisors and administrators to first deny must cease in order to prevent these and other unacceptable practices from taking place in the skilled nursing facility. A hidden camera should not be necessary to expose some of the ills "viewed from inside." The need for the ombudsman becomes more inevitable. In good medical management, we treat "risk factors" to prevent serious illnesses and to ensure the health and well-being of our patients. I view the exclusive attendance by young men of the personal hygiene care of female clients/patients as a needless "risk factor" conveniently created by administrators and supervisors; this practice should be treated as a "risk factor." Such action in no way reflects on the integrity of caregivers; it protects them and the administration in this litigious environment. Remember! "A stitch in time saves nine."

COUNTRIES OF ORIGIN: I found some correlation in the attitudes of caregivers with the countries of origin, though not statistically tested. Of those interviewed who worked for home care agencies and independent contractors, there were some correlation with work performance and countries of origin.

Job Designation and Countries of Origin:

1. Nursing Supervisor: Four directors of services, U.S. born and trained. Responsibilities, to oversee the job performance of home care workers

2. Nursing Consultant: One consultant U.S. born and trained. Responsibilities, to confirm and verify the medical/nursing status of applicants for Long Term Insurance benefits.

3. Staff Nursing: RN and LPN, most of whom were born and trained in the Philippines and the United Kingdom/and Caribbean. The proportion of staff trained outside the United States varied by location of institutions.

4. Social Service: Three director of services, U.S. born and trained. Responsibilities, to direct the Social Service department and its related functions.

5. Physical therapists: Six therapist (Philippine) born and trained. Eight U.S. born and trained. Responsibilities to evaluate and carry out therapy on eligible clients/patients in their homes.
Occupational therapist: Two therapists U.S. born and trained. Responsibilities, to evaluate and carry out therapy on eligible clients/patients in their homes.

6. Speech therapist: Four U.S. born and trained. Responsibilities, to evaluate and training of patients with speech and swallowing disorders.

7. Caregivers: These constitute a majority of those interviewed, (26)

    Countries of Origin:

    Jamaica, W.I.

    The Republic of The Philippines

    The Republic of Haiti

    The former British West Indian colonies

    The Republic of Guyana. Republic of Ghana. Republic of Chili. Brazil the United States.

It is important to note that these were random observations and not statistically tested.

Home care at the hands-on level (responsible for bathing, toileting, grooming, dressing, feeding, bed-mobility) was dominated by immigrants and minority workers, many of whom were from the Republic of Haiti, the Philippines and from the former British Caribbean Islands. Many of the professional staff (nurses, physical therapists, licensed practical nurses) came from the Philippines. Many of the higher administrative staff were born in the United States. I have been able to interview only a small number of U.S.-born African American, including three ward clerks. The number of U.S.-born workers, at any given institution, varied from location to location, with larger numbers further away from metropolitan areas. This question arose: Where are the native African American applicants when the unemployment rate is reportedly highest among members of this group? I arrived at a presumptive conclusion after talking to a community-based advocate, a clergyman, a social worker, and an unemployed African American, looking for work for nearly a year.

The unemployed asked bluntly, "Would you work for $7.75 an hour and have to provide your own meals. I would have to spend money. I don't have to do this."

At $9 an hour, working eight hours a day, a worker will earn $72 a day, $360 a week. A husband and wife in this pay bracket will earn $720 a week. When child care, transportation, meals, rent, and/or mortgage payments are deducted, only those of certain persuasion would continue to believe these are living wages. Under these circumstances, I have empathy with many African American and white Native American home care workers who may entertain some feeling of entitlement to a livable wage scale. I have no issues with their feeling of entitlement under these conditions. The reasoning for such disparity in living wages, which precludes some African Americans and some white Americans from accepting these low-paying jobs, is beyond the scope of this publication and would require in-depth studies to adequately elucidate. Some may argue with conviction and some justification that the pie is big enough for all who labor to have at least a taste, but the slices will have to be cut more proportionately. These advocates cite the disparity in earnings, "the pay scale of CEOs in the health care industrial complex, and ask, "Why should I work for wages which cannot sustain my needs as a human being, especially as an American-born citizen? The reasoning for their discontent is: "My slice is smaller or nonexistent because your slice is disproportionately too big." This inequity has gained the attention of the government, hence the 80/20 rule to establish a sense of fairness and equity. Yet the cry of government intervention is loud and clear by those who insist on maintaining the status quo. There is no doubt that government intervention, the Affordable Care Act, a case in point, will be inevitable and appropriate when greed dominates and the perspicacity of decision makers become blunted by sheer selfishness and arrogance.

During the interview, another revelation was the marginal socioeconomic status of many health care workers from foreign countries. The question I posed, how is it that these workers are offered the same low-scale wages and seem to be attracted to these jobs? Simplistic reasoning and answers to very complex and difficult situation do not always provide adequate explanation. Foreign-born workers, especially recent immigrants, are attracted to these often thankless low-pay jobs because of necessity. They have few alternatives and may not be eligible for some of the existing social umbrellas to which their American-born counterparts are entitled. However, the advantage the new immigrant enjoys has also to do with the level of their social and domestic environment prior to migration. For many immigrants, earning a regular wage is a welcomed change, even at the prevailing pay scale; Their needs are few and less demanding demanding than the American-born worker, who may consider an automobile a necessity; he also considers a television a necessity. These needs, real or contrived, make it virtually impossible for the American-born worker to accept the minimum and subminimum wages paid by many health care employers.

One of the probabilities is the immigrant worker may be accustomed to living in a smaller and more congested living quarters occasionally six or more individuals in one room. This becomes the norm and at significant savings when each individual contributes a small portion toward the total cost of living. This practice may be transported to their new domicile. This brings to mind the deplorable conditions in the Republic of Haiti following the 2002 earthquake disaster. Further, the immigrant worker will procure a bicycle and ride the one mile distance to his workplace. The automobile becomes a necessity for the American-born worker, whereas the foreign-born regards it as a luxury, certainly not a need. It is small wonder that many foreign-born workers are able to sustain themselves with marginal minimal wages, while their American counterparts find it near impossible to survive.

The socio-environmental conditions experienced by many recent immigrants may also have contributed to their ability to live with less and thus able to cope with what is in fact a very marginal wage scale. When I lectured one care worker, who had lived in the United States for three years, about the need for frequent hand washing, she promptly replied, "I don't want to waste your water."

I asked her, "Don't you wash your hands after toileting in your native country?"

She tersely replied, "We don't have running water where I lived. We don't even have sink. Where are we going to wash hands?"

This may seem shocking to many American workers. I was not surprised and the reason I asked the question was to hear it directly from the worker. My recent tour of some foreign countries as a volunteer clinician has confirmed this kind of "socioeconomic" enclaves where some of these emigrants have lived.

In the poorest American household, there are some facilities for basic social needs. There are differences in the quality of services rendered by health care workers based on the country of origin. This observation is not without some merit and has caused some employers to preclude the employment of applicants from certain countries. Some administrators have confirmed this practice. Looking at the ethnic makeup at some institutions supports this conclusion. The registered nursing (RN) staff, licensed practical nursing (LPN) staff, and nursing support staff were predominantly from the Republic of the Philippines at one institution. This required no statistical analysis to confirm; it was very apparent. Nursing aides at this institution were principally from the Republic of Haiti and the former British Caribbean colonies. I noted a similar trend in the United Kingdom as a medical student. Many of the registered nurses were from the Irish republic.

My experience with home care workers from one country had been a disaster until the arrangement was changed and workers from another country were employed. I found one worker intruding into my privacy, invading my closed desk, and reading my correspondence then lied about it; this correspondence was about a former worker about whom I had written the agency. During a later conversation, she was able to mention the name and address of this worker whom she had never met, never knew, and had the temerity to contact this worker based on the information she had obtained from my correspondence.

"A good liar should have a good memory"—this was not the case. The very worker after her attention was called to a dirty dish on which she was serving a client took umbrage and, without adequate notice, quit the job, leaving her dependent client stranded. I became very distrustful of this worker whom I believed had some pressing emotional problems. Her personal experiences were always grandiose in an environment where home sales were depressed and many homes abandoned—"My friend sold their home for $1.5 million." Another friend was paying $30,000 in school taxes. These are the employees that one must keep under surveillance. On one occasion, when I looked in to see the care she was giving my patient, she had the audacity to tell me "Why don't you take a walk?" Her departure was a blessing in disguise; it was like the absence of an intractable headache, unabated even with codeine. The fact that she was an independent contractor made it almost impossible to find a quick replacement. Such is the dilemma when one takes on an independent contractor. A health care agency would have found a replacement within a reasonable time.

Another worker from the same *country* assured me that she would be on the job on the following morning without fail. She never showed up and never called; imagine a dependent person without any assistance, not even to prepare breakfast. Another worker desperate to work from the same area suggested that the client should use her credit card and purchase a cot, place it in her living room to provide her a sleeping quarter so that she may start working ASAP. Needless to say, she was not hired.

These reports were unfortunate and came from workers from the same country; none knew the other worker. The temptation to draw negative conclusion is strong. Unless this can be statistically demonstrated, it has to be viewed as coincidental and probably irrelevant. But if you are an employer, would you take a chance for a dependent client? Yet some have reported excellent service from workers from those very countries. I have strong convictions that geographic domicile of applicants for certain home care positions could serve as an indicator of the success or failure of an employee. One home care worker told me that she did not like to work for black people because "they treat you like a servant."

After questioning her intensely, I concluded that she expected from the black employer/client a level of treatment which was inconsistent with her job description, a health care worker (caregiver). She was offended that she was not allowed to eat with other family members. She was asked to wear her uniform after she arrived for work one morning with a low-cut blouse with breasts partly exposed as though modeling for a magazine. Her real problem, in my view, was one of entitlement. I also extracted from her the fact that she did not eat with family members of the white client under her care, which she accepted as a matter of course. Her problem was also one of faulty perception of realities. It was difficult to fathom what she expected.

I reminded her, "You were employed to take care of the needs of a sick and disabled person, not to be his spouse or his 'lady in residence.'" I saw no offense by being excluded from having meals with the family. Perhaps that is the time for social and family engagement and for discussion of personal family matters which are of no interest to any health care worker, white or black. What's wrong with wearing uniform? You are required to wear one working in many institutions, whether you're black or white. She clearly showed a double standard in her expectation, forgetting that she was hired to perform the task of helping the disabled and to treat the person respectfully, not to be adopted as a family member. Many complaints and expressions of dissatisfaction were registered by clients and their family members regarding care and treatment given by caregivers. So much so, one is hard pressed to conclude on which side of the equation lies the imbalance. Whenever anyone charged with the care and responsibility for a disabled person commits a verbal or physical abuse or abandonment of such person, they should be made to defend such. In this context, assault may include abusive behavior, threats without the use of physical force.

THE I KNOW SYNDROME: The health care dilemma may also be exacerbated by problems caused by home care workers, especially the recent arrivals from foreign countries. Many of these workers are placed into social/domestic environments which are completely alien to them. Their pride often prevents them from admitting their lack of knowledge or savvy in performing simple tasks we take for granted. These tasks, however, may be essential for the care of their clients. To cover up their deficiencies in knowledge and/or training, many of them have given the same "knee-jerk" response to questions which portend to their knowledge: "I know! I know! I know!" I have also observed that the more repetitious the answer, the less they seem to understand. I have coined the "I-Know Syndrome" for the purposes of this book.

In medicine, a syndrome is often expressed as a series of signs and symptoms which characterize a disease process. The diabetic syndrome is characterized by polydipsia (excessive thirst and quest for water), polyphagia (excessive quest for food, especially carbohydrates), and polyuria (excessive urination).

This classic diabetic syndrome brings to mind a friend, a dental practitioner. Whenever I visited his office socially or professionally, he would produce a box with at least half a dozen jelly donuts and devoured most of them. His penchant for jelly donuts intrigued me because until then I had not seen nor eaten this concoction. His frequent visits to the men's room and the pitcher of water at his desk were also alarming to me. No one, including himself, knew that he was a diabetic, even though the syndrome (polyuria, polyphagia, and polydipsia) was "written on the wall," until he suddenly ended up with a diabetic coma and kidney shutdown. He was stricken, slumped in his car on his way home from his office, and taken to the emergency room by EMS/police.

Why did I single out "I know! I know!" as a syndrome worthy of mention in relation to home care? I have found with few exceptions that home care workers, with the arduous and often thankless task of caring for the sick and disabled, will seldom admit their lack of knowledge in many aspects of care; this includes the use of simple or complex utilities, fixtures in the home, or even procedures in the personal care of their charge. This is a very serious flaw and could result in disastrous consequences to the client and the home care worker.

A very interesting consistency was unfolded in my questioning; nearly all of the health care workers at some institutions fell in the following categories:

- Born outside the continental United States
- Formative education (elementary/high school) outside the continental United States
- Communication in fluent English marginal, not always easy to decipher
- Exposure to hygiene and sanitary codes not on par with practices in the United States

It was interesting to note that those who acknowledged their deficiencies were with college degrees or recognized certificates. The nurse/director (BS/RN) was quick to admit, "I don't know if occupational therapy comes into play, but as a stroke patient, she should have an OT consultation."

When she was asked to demonstrate the operation of a stove to the home care worker, she said, "I don't know anything about this brand. Do you have the manual?"

This approach contrasts sharply with that of the home care worker. I told her the clothes in the washing machine are to be washed, dried, and folded before she left for the evening, at eight o'clock. I then told her: "Let me show you how to use the washing machine before I leave."

The word machine had barely been spoken when she said "I know! I know!" almost as a defiance.

I left the apartment and returned within two hours, fully expecting the laundry to be washed, dried, and folded. When I opened the machine, the dirty clothes were staring at me, not laundered.

I asked: "Are you through washing the clothes?"

She said to me: "They still in the machine."

"What happened?" I asked.

She replied, "Me don't know how to turn on *you* machine," as though it was the fault of the machine.

"But you told me you knew how!"

She said, "You machine is different."

She probably had never used a washing machine in her life. This dialogue ended abruptly. I calmly turned on the machine. I was compelled to complete a task which was entirely her responsibility—another example of the I-Know Syndrome adding fuel to the home care dilemma.

The week end homecare worker was no better, it was the time when one wished for some lighter moments without stressful encounters with homecare workers. She avowed that she knew how to use the washing machine but didn't know how to turn it on. I took her at her words, but I demonstrated how to turn on the machine.

"Do you know the rest?" I asked.

"I know! I know!"

I left the apartment and returned within an hour. I was very pleased to hear the spinning cycle in operation and felt that she had refuted the theory of my I-know syndrome. But it then dawned on me that it was a rather short cycle for the machine. When I opened the machine, the syndrome was there in full operation. It was the spin/dry cycle but not a drop of water in the machine. She only knew how to start the machine as I had demonstrated but did not know how to turn on the water, another home care dilemma.

Family members or those supervising the care of the sick or disabled should make no assumption about the knowledge or experience of caregivers without concrete evidence. This is especially true with regard to the application of devices, such as prostheses (artificial limbs), braces, splints, etc. It also applies to preparation of meals. It must be remembered that caregivers, for the most part, are from environments which may be vastly different from yours; this fact significantly influences the way people operate within the same environment, even the perception of right and wrong. Few family members, clients, or administrators wish to confront this issue, although off-the-cuff remarks clearly indicate their deeper convictions. Their actions contradict their feeling. This contradiction reminds me of a story I've heard:

A very successful businessman entered a car dealership with two of his colleagues. They were showed several Mercedes, Cadillacs, BMWs, and Jaguars. After several hours of viewing and discussions, the businessman decided on the Jaguar and paid outright by check. As he was leaving, one salesman whispered to the other, "See that man with his friends? He just bought a Jaguar only because he's with his big-shot friends, but I believe, deep down in his heart, he knew he wanted a Caddy."

I returned from a grand round one Wednesday, having left our caregiver in charge of my spouse; she had been with us for over a month and had won our trust, even though having shown minor but significant flaws; no human being is perfect. When I noticed that my wife was unable to bend her right knee, and it would have been impossible to sit on the commode, which was required, I took a closer look. Our trusted caregiver had placed the brace backward so that the right knee was extended. The opening over the patella, which allowed free movement of the knee joint, was now covered, and the bands above and below the patella were reversed.

Several days after, the splint for the affected left wrist, specially fabricated to support a left wrist drop, was applied by the caregiver. To my surprise, she placed it so that the portion which was obviously contoured for the palm of the left hand and wrist was now incorrectly placed over the back of the unaffected right hand, a double-header. These and other faux pas were perfect examples of the I-know syndrome, which I must bring to your attention. However, these transgressions, I must confess, were relatively small when weighed against the enormous humanity and good will exhibited by many home care workers whose services are invaluable.

POTENTIAL PROBLEMS AND PROBLEMS: I would be remiss if I failed to alert you of the possibility of preexisting health problems affecting health care workers, especially home care workers who are directly recruited by clients or family members. These workers are usually selected based on recommendations by family or friends; they seldom if ever, undergo any physical examination prior to employment and could pose some risk to their employer, especially those who are Mantoux positive (TB-positive skin test). For those contracted and employed by institutions (hospitals, nursing homes, long-term care facilities, group homes), some of the potential health problems are minimized. Many institutions have facilities for health screening. Some workers may require additional tetanus, diphtheria, prophylactic inoculations. Health care agencies, which are responsible for placement of workers, also screen potential employees, but their policies appear to be less exacting, and they cover mainly education and background check. One reason may be that the demand for trained health care workers is a tight one, hence some agencies may forego their rigid testing requirements in order to maintain a list of potential employees. When several agencies are located in a small catchment area, there is greater competition for potential workers and testing requirements are relaxed.

There is little doubt that immigrant workers, recent arrivals, present greater health risk than native-born Americans. Most American-born children are required by local public health codes to undergo certain basic health examinations and receive preventive care. Health codes and practices in many of the countries from which immigrants migrate are nonexistent or wantonly ineffective. I found children in a number of countries grown to be adults and parents without ever having any of the tests or inoculations we take for granted.

When entering into independent contract (direct contract between client and caregiver), especially when health risk may be a concern, the following are Important Considerations: Inquire about the length of time worker has lived in the United States, the country of origin, and recent overseas travel. Immigrants from certain countries are more likely to have or to have been exposed to certain diseases. You have a right to know this before you employ.

A twenty-two-year-old female patient I examined for unexplained weight loss told me, "Doctor, I think I have worms."

"How do you know?" I inquired.

She said: "I see one coming through my nose."

This may have been an unusual case, but it happens. This young woman was a potential immigrant and certainly a carrier. Inquire whether applicant has any prior experience in a U.S. hospital or hospital in their country of origin; these employees may have had prior health screening. Contact the institution to confirm prior employment and any record of prior testing.

POTENTIAL PROBLEMS: Inquire about any recent hospitalization or doctor's visit and reasons. Perhaps the most efficient way to obtain these information without appearing to be intrusive is to construct a questionnaire well in advance and request that applicant complete the routine application form. The protection of your loved ones and yourself should be paramount. Any reasonable inquiry into present or past relevant health issues should be fair game. If there is any overt resistance on the part of the applicant, I assure you there is reason for doubts. Inquire about ability to perform reasonable assisted transferring of clients. Home caregivers may at some time be required to do some lifting. Clients with varying degrees of weakness may have to be lifted during transfer activities. Inquire about history of any musculoskeletal disorders, any low back pain or disc problems.

A line must be drawn between a companion and a caregiver/aide, and this must be unequivocally defined and understood in advance of employment. A companion's role is very limited. He/She is expected to provide only human conversational stimulation, to protect the client from self-injury and in some cases assist in feeding, grooming, and dressing. Contrasts between the health care agencies and the independent contractor should also be made known. Companions may also prepare light meals and clean and tidy the client's immediate surroundings.

Most health care agencies function very much like employment agencies; in principle, they are paid by clients or family members. The rate charged by the agency is then apportioned between the caregiver and the agency. Example: It is not uncommon for a health care agency charging the client $20 per hour of work then pays the health care worker/aide $9 per hour. I am told some agencies may pay as much as $12 per hour. The remainder goes to the health care agency toward administrative and other costs. The independent contractor has no middleman. Whatever fee is contracted goes directly to the caregiver.

Under these circumstances, they often contract for smaller hourly rates than with health care agencies but receive a significantly higher hourly rate than what is paid by the agencies. Factors such as insurance and Medicare payments are the responsibilities of caregiver. These differences, including advantages and disadvantages, are dealt with in greater detail in appropriate publications and should be consulted.

Problems which occur in your homes may be considered small and insignificant, but cumulatively, they become costly and a source of irritation. On the first day on the job, one care worker entered the kitchen holding her empty cup firmly. Her first question to me was "Where is the tea bags?" I was so stunned that instinctively I began looking in the cupboard for tea bags. She then tersely said to me, "I look there already." She did not last very long. Was she here to drink tea or to work?

Some common infractions are oblivious to many caregivers as a consequence of their past environment. This lack of awareness compounds the problem and makes it more difficult to correct. I have stressed the need to establish ground rules before an applicant is employed, these are repeated on the first day of his /her employment and thereafter, they establish jurisdictional control and responsibilities. It should be made crystal clear that a caregiver is employed primarily to fulfill the needs of the client/infirmed and at the pleasure of the client or his family. The methods used in performing her duties are the prerogative of the experienced caregiver, provided no harm is done to the client or the surroundings. Full control of your home should remain with you, the client or family members, unless otherwise expressly relegated. This prerogative should not be abdicated, except under the most extreme circumstances, if your home environment is to retain your unique characteristics. Always keep in mind that many caregivers may come from environments which markedly differ from your own. They may instinctively make changes to reflect a surrounding alien to you.

As my wife improved, she began to observe changes and infractions which she disliked but preferred me calling them to the attention of the caregivers. She was very mindful of the fact that she was the recipient of their benevolence and good will. She was not prepared to be the object of their anger. "Let the doctor do this, he is always prognosticating." Further, I had established the dubious reputation, not as a consultant physician but as an army sergeant. I was not smiling over this unwanted promotion. It was not a compliment by any stretch of the imagination. Although her vision was somewhat impaired by the stroke, she called my attention to three large circular imprints on the wall recently painted. As I looked more closely, there were three large areas of grease or oil from the oil-saturated hair of our caregiver. She used the wall as her pillow while snoozing, sitting in a chair. Our attempt to remove them only resulted in erosion of the paint and necessitated a touching up with paint. The caregiver was unimpressed. When this was brought to her attention she said: "It's only a little grease mark."

Similarly, the faucet in the bath was so abused by forcefully tunting off, it had to be changed or repaired three times within several months. Of these infractions, no one knew who caused them, though the caregivers are the only users. When the rubber connection of the shower head was busted because the outer protecting metal was broken, I just refused to have it replaced. I had enough.

Expressions and the use of words should not be ignored, they may be the cause of serious miscommunication. A patient/client suddenly became diaphoretic and listless. The caregiver, in her attempt to revive the patient, excitedly exclaimed, "Get a rag! Get a rag! And wipe her face!" For a moment, those around her were bewildered. "What is she talking about?" It is well known that in this environment (US), one's face is never wiped with rags under any circumstances. Rags are pieces of waste cloth used for mopping the floor or cleaning. Fortunately, there was no breach in safety of this patient/client because no rags were available nor applied. A wet towel was appropriately applied. This caregiver had no intention using a floor mop to wipe the face of her charge. The use of water by some home caregivers was always excessive and wasteful. This occurred frequently with those who had been exposed to running water for a relatively short time. I do believe that some of these excesses were inadvertent and reflected the formative domicile of those workers.

Another location for abuse were doors. Caregivers would use the wooden frame around the doors for closing; as a consequence of this practice, the painted frames around the door and adjacent to the doorknobs were blackened by the soiled hands of caregivers. The most alarming aspect of these problems, they never perceive them as problems worthy of correction. I see some of their actions as vandalism. They cause home care to be more costly and prohibitive, even with assistance from insurance carriers. I have observed supplies (soap, gloves, paper, cleaning detergents) being used in ways which can only be described as reckless. On one occasion, I threatened to deduct cost of any damage to the house from their paychecks in an attempt to curb this extravagance.

It is relatively easy for some caregivers to transform their new environment, your home, into a place unfit to live, unless there is close and rigid supervision. Such supervision may best be carried out by one who is familiar with acceptable norms and standards practiced in your home. The same principles may be applied to the skilled nursing care environment.

I equate this problem with caregivers to carrying sticky chewing gum on the sole of your shoes. As you travel from one room to another, the gum remains fixed under your shoes. You only get rid of it by discarding your shoes or scraping off the gum. I think of the gum as entrenched bad habits and behavior (assaults to clients when not being observed, yelling at patients/clients who cannot understand your thick foreign accent, abandoning your charge abruptly and unattended in the midst of toilet care because "my shift is over") I attribute this inhumane behavior to poor orientation of caregivers or a flaw in character and one who is unsuited for the kind of work he/she is committed to do. This is tantamount to walking out in the middle of an appendectomy because the surgeon's shift is over. I have no empathy for these workers. They knew the nature of the work for which they were hired. When they accepted the job, they also accepted the responsibilities and obligations. They could not have assumed that they were on their way to Harvard or Princeton University. This type of worker will continue with this flawed practice wherever he/she goes and, like the chewing gum, may have to be scraped off or discarded.

I walked into my wife's hospital room at eight o'clock one morning. There were discarded gloves, used paper towels, and empty intravenous plastic bags scattered about the floor not far from the waste bin. I could not figure out why all these discarded materials were on the floor in proximity of the waste bin. I donned a pair of gloves and picked up all of them and placed them into the waste bin.

After a few minutes, in comes the "prima donna," the aide (PCA). She introduced herself and stated that she was about to take blood sample for analysis. After completing her task, she threw the blood-stained sponge on the floor near to the waste bin. She then went into the bathroom, washed her hands, then again threw the wet paper towel on the floor next to the waste bin. I then thought I should say something. After all, it was my wife's room, for which I paid hundreds of dollars each day. Where are the supervisors?

I said to her, "Excuse me! I believe you have dropped something on the floor, you dropped three pieces of discarded materials on the floor."

She said to me, "Don't worry about it, they would clean it up later." Later meant several hours wait.

I reminded her that I was paying for a clean room. I then called the nurse in charge who picked up the materials and placed them into the waste bin. She then said to me, "They are not nurses, they are aides," as if to dissociate those actions from what are expected of nurses.

I had to conclude that this worker, who apparently was a recent immigrant by her speech, was intent on deliberately transforming the hospital room to look like hospital rooms in her native country where trash was perhaps discarded anywhere on the floor. The RN who picked up the trash did nothing to educate her. In my exasperation, I asked myself, "Where do these people come from?" It also indicates the difficulties institutions experience in recruiting, training, and retaining workers of quality for the important task of patient care.

This problem also extends to other areas of responsibility for the immigrant and domestic worker. The woman who cleans my office came into my office in tears, sobbing that she had been fired. She was accused of not vacuuming and dusting the office on a daily basis. Her supervisor had placed pieces of paper on the floor which were never swept up nor vacuumed for several days. She said: "Doc, the place ain't dirty." She insisted that the office was clean, yet bits and pieces of paper littered the floor. Shelves and cabinets with dust were evidence to the contrary. I reminded her that her contract and job description called for daily vacuuming and dusting and that she failed to do these tasks. She was subsequently rehired after counseling. This incident also supports my view for a job description for each health care worker. It provides structure for the employee. It is an important feature in management because it also provides an instrument to address work covered and by whom.

I would hope that she learned a lesson. She would not be rehired a second time. This woman was the victim of her native environment where dust must be overwhelming to be recognized as dust.

Some problems created by caregivers may have serious medical consequences as the case of a compressed urine bag. A Foley catheter was connected to a thigh-bag reservoir which was emptied periodically, a simple procedure requiring only common sense and two hands to carry out. After four hours had elapsed and there was no urine in the bag, although the patient was on IV fluids, I asked the nurse to check. The caregiver had placed the collecting bag under the patient's thigh then connected the Foley catheter to the bag. The weight of patient's thigh completely compressed the bag that no urine entered but instead backed up into the catheter. Fortunately, the length of the catheter acted as a reservoir and prevented urine from backing up into the patient's bladder. When she returned after several hours and found the bag empty, she remarked, "Eh! Eh! This thing ain't working! I got to call the nurse." I was reluctant to intervene but then decided to go against my initial instinct and explained to her that the weight of patient's thigh had compressed the bag.

One may reasonably dismiss these problems as coincidence; however, when there is a pattern, as I have observed, other conclusions have to be drawn. It is tempting to ascribe these problems as being peculiar to the recent immigrant worker, but I do not have enough evidence to draw such conclusion.

The paucity of U.S.-born citizens who work as caregivers, either as home care providers or institution-based, deserve attention not covered in this publication, although alluded to in other sections of this book. Though the purpose of this book is not intended to offer remediation or solutions, I have offered a few practical and easily followed rules and dogmas for dealing with some of the inevitable problems encountered in home care delivery.

Clients and family members must seize upon the initial orientation period for caregivers to make their case. They must make known their principles and expectations. I would go a step further and enumerate the common and frequent problems caused by the caregivers, many of which are mentioned throughout this publication. A copy of your listing should then be given to prospective employees after a full discussion of each of your concern; this should be signed by employees who retain a copy. My greatest concern relates to those caregivers who function in the home environment; those working in institutions often receive more structured training and better supervision.

The problems in health care delivery are enormous and varied. Institutions, health care agencies, and individual contractors must share responsibility for some of the problems I have observed. Most applicants interviewed when asked why they have chosen health care delivery as their vocation replied: "I like the kind of work. I like to work with people who are disabled to get them back on their feet. I am glad to know I helped someone who can't help himself." Of the eighteen interviewed, only one stated, "I need the money, and this is the quickest job I could get." That was her motivation for accepting the job. I came to the conclusion that money was her primary interest. In fact, with their job skills and their level of communication, most of them would be hard pressed finding employment elsewhere.

In spite of their claims, there was a disconnect between their stated experience during the interview and their actual job performance, especially in relation to their attitude toward patients/clients under their care. Patients had been left unattended, half dressed, and partially cleaned (toileted) because the caregiver's shift was over before she completed her care. Night clothing was tossed on the bed of a patient/client who was activity-of-daily-living (ADL) dependent, with the almost intimidating assertion, "Here is your night clothes. I have to go, my shift over." Nurses have to complete their reports and hand over their charges to the relieving shift. Physicians have to complete their histories and physicals on a new patient, regardless of the time involved. It was clear that the professional staff always showed a greater sense of responsibility.

So what influences such callous attitude toward the sick and disabled by the very aides whose stated desire was to help the sick and disabled? I feel a sense of personal hurt and anger for the victims of abuse who are petrified to utter a word of disapproval for fear of revenge. Where are the advocates for these victims? Yet there are unions and other advocates for the workers. Only workers have rights?

I have seen patient/client with incipient skin breakdown over the coccyx (tailbone) and their heels who were in great discomfort, sitting in a wheelchair with an unyielding seat for about twelve hours. When I personally intervened to have a patient transferred to her bed with air mattress, the nurse in charge could not find anyone who was responsible for her care to assist with the transfer. "They are on their break," he said.

"All of them at the same time? Who is in charge?" I asked.

I then volunteered to assist. The patient was then transferred to her bed by the nurse and an aide who later appeared on the scene.

Experience has led me to conclude that the orientation training of new workers and the supervision process at a number of institutions were seriously flawed. The aides, for the most part, seem not to fully understand the reasons for which they were employed. Supervisors seem to be nonexistent and/or afraid to supervise. Not knowing who are on break during your watch seems inexcusable. Many of the answers to these difficult questions relate to training and the selection process. Training sessions should not be monologues with one speaker dominating the process and speaking only in the first person singular. The caregivers should be allowed and encouraged to fully participate, especially in relation to issues and their work expectations. Some of the more unpleasant aspects of employment should also be presented; these should not be swept under the rug. They should always be reminded that they will be serving clients who are senile, incontinent of urine and feces, and these clients/patients have to be cleaned and sanitized completely, when these conditions occur during their charge. These are the sticky issues which have not been well explained nor fully understood by many caregivers. Perhaps equally important, caregivers must be constantly reminded that wearing a pair of gloves is not always a substitute for regular hand washing. Most of those I have observed do not wash their hands as often as they should and wear the same pair of gloves from one room to another.

It is not enough to have high-level administrative meetings. Administration needs to know what goes on at the other side of the coin and to hear directly from those who are in the line of duty, the hands-on caregivers. A very common complaint against administrators and supervisors by both employees and patients/clients: "Nothing will change. They don't listen. They don't care." My experience as a clinical administrator convinces me that administrators will listen, they do care, and they often consider complaints which appear to have merits. We have come to the realization that hospitals/institutions exist because of patients/clients; when people stop using these facilities, they fold up. These hard facts compel management to be more responsive to the needs of the people they serve. Government agencies also expect a fair percentage of the earnings from patients go toward patients' care, the 80/20 rule.

Some caregivers have complained after they were hired that the work is difficult and the pay is not enough. I find this as their justification for patients' neglect or abuse (physically or mentally) totally unacceptable and unwarranted. I do understand that the pay scale for many caregivers is marginal, but each worker is briefed when he/she applied for employment. They know what the work entails at the wages they agreed upon.

Many caregivers are aware that their clients/patients have varying degrees of ADL deficits and others are entirely dependent. It is, therefore, reasonable to assume that the job requirements and responsibilities are understood. They know that their clients are frail; it is not as though they are expected to perform like members of a high school football team in a physical fitness program. Any proven serious infraction or abuse of a client should result in the immediate suspension of their services and/or legal adjudication. All employees should be well aware of these expectations prior to their employment. This disclosure should be the responsibility of the employer. It must be remembered that the clients/patients are at the mercy of the caregivers. Many of the patients interviewed were afraid of reprisals and would not complain of abuse or serious neglect; these have to be detected by the patient's advocate, supervisory nurse, or social worker. In handling these complaints, institutions must keep in mind that they exist solely for the benefit of the clients/patients they have the privilege to serve, not for their caregivers or the administrative boards.

VIRTUES AND CONTRADICTIONS Much has been written about caregivers, especially the home care workers. Many negative experiences were reported and documented in this book; verification of the events indicate that many of them had some validity. Some were so outlandish that termination of services was effected.

In balance, I have had the pleasure of receiving commendable reports about a number of home care workers who dispel the negative reports about a few undesirable workers. When I relate my good fortune to prospective employers, one question frequently asked: "How can you determine in advance of employment who would be a good home care worker, and how can you predict which institution would best serve the needs of my loved ones?" For the most part, it is trial and error, but I have determined that a questionnaire was a very useful and desirable instrument to make this determination. It is seen by applicants as routine. It elicits the answers you need to make your decision and does not seem to be intrusive.

Experience has shown that there is some correlation with quality care and country of origin. It seems that workers from certain countries tend to be more abrasive, adamant, and confrontational. I have avoided these workers in the selection process and with good outcome. It is interesting to note that other employers have had similar experience. I have used the following guidelines in the selection process:

- The ability to communicate in the language of the client/patient is most important.
- The number of years in the United States and in home care services—those working in the service for over five years seem to show better outcome.

- Consistency in working with the same clients, working with the same family for an extended period, has indicated a measure of trust and stability.
- The age of the worker—younger workers were more likely to quit without advance notice. They were also more likely to report absent and being tardy, more likely to use their employment as a "stepping stone."
- The distance from place of employment and means of transportation—one worker who was always late, was always delayed at the railroad crossing, or because the battery of her car was dead. Someone else was always the cause of her tardiness. She never accepted personal responsibility for being late. Paradoxically, workers living furthest from workplace were usually on time.

Perhaps the best way to secure a reasonably satisfactory caregiver is by word of mouth, a recommendation by one who has had personal experience with the candidate, or recommendation by a caregiver who already has the reputation of competence and being trustworthy. This method has seldom failed to yield a good outcome.

To support *the* workers engaged in home health care and in appreciation of the important service they render to the community, the labor department has intervened on their behalf to collect funds from health care agencies due to workers.

According to the U.S. Department of Labor, the Fair Labor Standards Act (FLSA) requires that covered employees be paid at least the federal minimum wage of $7.75 for all hours worked (now increased) plus time and one half their rates. This includes commissions, bonuses, and incentive pay for hours worked beyond forty hours per week. In general, "hours worked" include all time an employee must be on duty or on the employer's premises or at any other prescribed place of work from the beginning of the first principal work activity to the end of the last principal work activity of the whole day. Additionally, the law requires that accurate records of employees' wages, hours, and other conditions of employment be maintained. The department finds nearly $275,000 in back wages due health care workers at one state-based home care service.

The virtues we find in many caregivers are often masked by the many infractions committed by a few bad apples tucked away in their midst. These undesirables should be exposed and removed from the roster of home care workers. All health care workers, however, should not be painted with one broad brush. One care worker reminded me that home care workers are reflection of the society in which we live. There was reasoned basis for his assertion; for if our society at large is corrupt, uncaring, and devoid of empathy, so would be the applicants from that society. This reasoning may also be extended to include doctors, lawyers, police, firemen, and members at large from that society. After all, these caregivers are not recruited from heaven.

Only the cynic would deny the valued services rendered by many caregivers, without which many of our loved ones may not enjoy that sought-after quality of life in their twilight years. One social worker related that "The home health care worker who took care of my dad saved my family." She explained that it was the caregiver who held the family together as no individual family member was able to do. Good and dedicated caregivers are difficult to replace because they are often called upon to take on lifesaving responsibilities especially when left alone to care for a family member. By the time a family member is summoned and arrives at the scene may be too late. A simple emergency may thus become a life-threatening catastrophe. It is difficult to comprehend how a human person could be spat upon and verbally abused yet carry out her assigned responsibilities with decorum and grace.

Caregivers, with few exceptions, work under conditions which few native-born Americans will tolerate and often at a pay scale which parallels poverty level, although employed full time. I observed with pain and disgust a patient receiving her morning care in bed. The caregivers were oblivious to her severely arthritic right knee. One grasped her right leg, the other her shoulder and attempted to turn the patient on her left side while the victim cried out for pain in the right knee. There was no attempt to roll the patient over in unison to limit or restrict the sudden and severe shock to her arthritic right knee that was already traumatized by the usual morning stiffness and pain. This patient/client may well have been your loved one. I hasten to mention that although the intervention described was unacceptable, I temper this with some understanding because of the background of the caregivers involved, having considered the training they may have received at that institution.

One caregiver, a recent immigrant having worked at that institution for just under a year, was disconnecting the plug from the wall socket. She held the long connecting cord and yanked the plug from the socket so that portion of the socket was removed. There was nothing gentle nor sensual in her action. The same worker was unperturbed that she had thrown the empty Foley bag on the floor rather than into the nearby waste bin. She even smiled as she looked in my direction.

My regrettable conclusion was her entire approach in turning the patient had little to do with her training, if any. There was no evil or uncaring intent or one without compassion. It was a mirror image of a tough, unrelenting background, and like the chewing gum stuck to the sole of her shoes and carried from institution to institution and patient to patient, she was completely unaware of the harm she was committing.

To exacerbate this dilemma, there was a problem with her ability to communicate. Yet, for her effort and willingness to attempt tasks which so many others refuse to do for the compensation she receives, I commend her. I also commend those skilled, honorable, and dedicated care workers for the exceptional service they perform. The health care system would be in great jeopardy without the services of our health care workers/aides.

I asked one caregiver, a nurse, "Why is it that so many Caribbean-born seem attracted to the health care vocation?" This question had haunted me for some time, and I was determined to get "an inside view." She was hesitant at first, but after she was assured that the information given was for a book on the delivery of health care and that no names nor workplaces would be mentioned, she spoke freely and without prompt.

I like doing what I do. I could have done teaching or something else, have better hours, better pay, and security, but it is not the same as caring for the sick. We from the Caribbean are more caring, even up to the sanitary needs of our patients. There are some people (referring to another ethnic group) who wouldn't even tidy their own sick family. I believe we have more compassion for people and more patience in dealing with them. Take a mother with four or five children in the Caribbean, she would never think of hiring someone to care for her children, even if she can afford. I see people here with one child and not working. They have to hire someone to take care of that child, them too lazy and have no love, no caring to take care of that child, especially when it comes to cleaning and toileting their own. I don't understand it. You would think that after carrying that child for nine months, you would want to cherish that child in every way possible until he is old enough to be on his own. I think our love for people was passed on to us. It is part of our culture. You cannot buy it with money because we had no money. We have something bigger than money, but you cannot see it, you cannot spend it, but you can feel it. It is love and compassion. If one don't like to take care of her own child, do you think that child would want to take care of you in your old age? The problem in this country, I find that people, especially people with money, are too busy, even when they have nothing to do, them have no time to love and care for their elders. That is why you find so many of us doing this kind of work. We care about people.

Her expressions may be an oversimplification, but they properly expressed her deep conviction and emotions. This respondent was born in the Caribbean and received most of her formative education in one of the former British Caribbean territories. She received her nurse's training in the New York area and had done nursing care for most of her working experience. She is now retired but enjoys doing per diem coverage.

My interview of most caregivers from the Caribbean reflected the same sentiment, but my observation of care given to their clients did not entirely support this view. The inclusion of ethnicity as a criterion in determining the quality care given at an institution seemed irrelevant.

To give a balanced view of the extent and quality of care given by home caregivers, the people whom I have come to regard as heroes, I include this *open letter* of invitation and recommendation, transcript from my condo bulletin with names changed:

A few years back, my cousin had a stroke and was not good. She was also around ninety years old. Thanks to super care, she lasted several more years.

Her children found a super caring lady that I call really a saint. She cared for my cousin for several years and was so unbelievable, caring, and attentive to an unhappy older lady. My cousin was thankful for the loving care received from Mona over the time. When my cousin was in pain and not the nicest, Mona was always as sweet and caring and simply understood the pain of my cousin. Mona always acted the same, peaceful angelic care. Much later, when my cousin required hospice, they could not believe that there were *no bedsores* anywhere on my cousin. Mona used to rub down my cousin with ointments, etc. after bathing her, also that she and the room, etc. were spotless. There is so much more I could say, but you can always ask me if you want more. After my cousin died, my neighbors then needed someone like Mona, and I recommended her to them. They told similar stories about Mona, about her level constant caring and love. They could not understand how Mona put up with it all.

Mona is originally from the islands. She lives in the Bronx but prefers to do live-in care. To my knowledge, she does not drive and uses public transportation. Hence, she prefers live-in during the workdays. She is extremely strong and gentle. And very important is her honesty. Totally extremely honest and trustworthy. She is also extremely religious, not Catholic, but in her "sitting time," she is usually reading the

Bible and praying. To me, she is like having a private Sister Therese.

BLACK VERSUS WHITE CAREGIVERS: A commonly expressed opinion that minority workers, workers of color, were more caring and showed greater empathy for the elderly clients/patients was not supported by my experience. My observation was limited to segments of two states. A very different picture may emerge in other parts of the country. In several institutions, where there were large numbers of white caregivers and several black residents, preference was frequently shown for certain white caregivers, who were said to be gentler, kinder, and less abrasive. Many have read or viewed the report where the daughter of an elderly African American gentleman having suspected abusive treatment of her father had a camera installed in the home. The camera was placed in the room where her father was virtually confined to bed, requiring assistance for most of his needs. The physical abuse inflicted upon this elderly gentleman by his caregiver was caught on camera; it was merciless, with assault and battery; this worker was arrested and subsequently prosecuted. This worker was of the same ethnicity as her charge. No compassion was shown to this gentleman because of their common ethnicity. What I viewed would have been unacceptable for any domestic animal. If white caregivers were found guilty of such abusive conduct, it would more likely be reported as "racial abuse." When the black/workers of color are accused of similar abusive conduct, they are characterized as heartless, evil people. It is regrettable that the stigma of this misdeed by the white worker is automatically characterized as racial abuse when race may never have entered the mind of the accused; he/she may just have been a heartless, cruel individual who happened to be white. Such stereotypes on both sides of the spectrum are unwarranted, very dangerous, and inciting. These misdeeds will continue because of the knee-jerk reaction of denial by those in place to make changes. You cannot correct or change what is not recognized.

People drawn to serve in the delivery of health care as their choice and vocation are more likely to serve their clients/patients with humanity. Those who enter because it is the only job they could find or able to do are more likely to be intemperate in dealing with seniors. Many of these individuals are forced into health care delivery by necessity, having no interest in care of the elderly and disabled.

The parents of a recent graduate of an offshore medical school told me, "My older son is a lawyer. We had to have a doctor in the family." Another medical graduate who was literally pushed through medical school by his mother, and ultimately graduated, now works at his father's establishment, a field completely unrelated to medicine. These are examples of "vocations of convenience," which are sometimes detested to an extent that those they serve become the victim of "a square peg in a round hole."

When people are forced into vocations or occupations they detest or have no interest in them, their dislike soon influences their work performance; they may show hostility, emotional and/or physical detachment for the tasks they perform. I have seen workers abruptly terminating routine care because the clock pointed to 5:00 p.m., time to quit; fortunately, these cases are few and exceptional. On the other hand, I have witnessed those who literally have to be taken off their tasks to have a meal. These are the dedicated professionals who have entered their professions to serve the needs of their clients/patients. They are seldom adequately compensated for their services.

HEALTH CARE LINKS/COMMUNICATION: We are linked by our ability to communicate. I heard numerous comments from family members of clients/patients who bitterly complained about the poor level of communication between caregivers and clients/patients.

One member said, "My mother is ninety-one and has osteoporosis. She didn't come here for physical therapy. She lived alone and now wants a place where people could talk to her. I don't understand half the things those aides say to her, neither does she."

This is the dilemma faced by institutions, caregivers, and their charge. It occasionally deteriorates into a shouting match when the caregiver tries to make herself understood to her charge who has a hearing loss superimposed on the inability to understand the caregiver who speaks her native language very poorly to say nothing about her ability to speak even broken English. Suspicion and disgust heighten when people are unwilling or unable to communicate in a common language in the health care environment. Perhaps, more importantly, the desired objectives and response are more difficult to achieve.

"You receive the urinal when you request the bed pan." There is no doubt that failure to communicate effectively invariably results in a fiasco. In many parts of the country, this dilemma is the rule rather than the exception, and institutions continue to have difficulties in recruiting caregivers who are able to communicate in a satisfactory manner with their clients/charge.

My college experience is a case in point: Fisher and Jaggat were roommates. Fisher was from Kentucky, and Jaggat was a recent arrival from one of the British Caribbean countries. Although they roomed together for several weeks, it became clear to me that they did not always fully understand each other. They got along very well and seemed reluctant and embarrassed to reveal that they did not always understand each other. Paradoxically, they were both from English-speaking countries. To "break the ice" and expose their apparent secret, I entered their room one morning with a mutual friend and jokingly asked Fisher to tell Jaggat that he was going to cut his throat. Without fanfare, Fisher, in his Kentucky brogue, said to Jaggat, "Jaggat! I'm going to cut your throat." With that said, I was expecting Jaggat to scramble out of the room or take cover under his bunk. I was amazed to see Jaggat, smiling broadly, said to Fisher, "OK! How nice!"

After I intervened and explained what Fisher had said, Jaggat was horrified with his answer and at the thought of near losing his life with his full consent. This is in fact a classic example of poor communication. However, this language barrier is not uncommon in the health care environment, especially when workers are hired through the health care agencies or hired directly by institutions. Individual contracts seem to make better choices. Many of these are workers who were recommended by others who have worked for the same family.

We are linked by our ability to communicate. To bridge or soften this dilemma in the delivery of care, there should be closer attention to a more reasonable communication skill during the selection process.

There should also be greater effort to train and recruit more members from the local community.

The low level of communication skill among caregivers was discussed with an administrator who was aware of the problem. It was agreed that improved communication would inevitably improve the standard of care by improving the social environment in which the infirmed must live. It must be remembered that these workers have more contact with clients/patients than other professional staff and certainly more than any administrator. Many suggestions were offered, including a more exacting selection process in which a simple English test is administered. It is my considered judgment that a large number of the caregivers at some facilities would fail to qualify for the task they now carry out. Administrators have reminded me that many institutions will not be able to function without the availability of these workers. Tuition incentive plan was also suggested where the worker does remedial studies in English; this was flatly rejected by a care worker who said, "I have a family to care for. I work from 7:00 p.m. to 7:00 a.m. at one job then from 8:00 a.m. to noon at another, sixteen hours a day. What time do I have to study English?"

It seems that most caregivers have structured themselves to the extent that any new commitment in time or money has to revolve around the priorities already in place. This fact bodes poorly for most of those who need remediation in the worst way, though I know of cases where the young worker seems content to spend her days playing games and other nonproductive endeavors instead of using that time pursuing some online course in basic grammar. It is a question of desire to improve oneself and motivation. You either have it or you don't.

Another suggestion was to have an instructor visit the institution once weekly for an hour of instructions. The question: "Who will pay the workers' expenses and for the instructor's time?" Incentive pay for improved communication skill in English was another option, but this would be costly for institutions and cumbersome to evaluate. It would cause more problems than it solves. The dilemma persists. There was no easy solution to a pressing problem.

It seems that with the urgent need for foot soldier (caregivers) in the health care industry, administrators have little interest in achieving communication skills for caregivers currently employed. They may hire anyone with two legs, two hands, who can get to work daily and on time.

The perennial problems in the delivery of health care are the demand for skilled trained workers, inadequate communication skills in many new immigrant workers, extravagant waste, and a gross compensation inequity for the work they do. If CEOs address the latter, there is fear that the compensation and other cushions they receive would be made a little bit harder for their established comfort level. I can well imagine the pain and suffering it would cause to reduce one's income from ten million a year to five million; this is a 50 percent reduction. How unconscionable! No one presumes that the worker's pay should rival that of CEOs. But surely, it should remove him from the poverty level. The lower echelon, the caregivers, was presumed to have greater tolerance for this kind of pain. Appreciation for their services was not met with equitable compensation for their labor, yet they represent the most important link in the chain of operation.

The importance of this link becomes apparent because the system only operates well as a chain. The CEOs, the highest paid, are the largest links of the chain. Their salaries, bonuses, stock options boggle the imagination and bewilder the rank and file. Paradoxically, the strength of the chain of operation does not relate to the largest link; it lies in the smallest and weakest link, the caregiver. This link must be strengthened if the system is to function as a chain because it represents the strength of the functional unit. If this link is ruptured, the entire operation ceases to function smoothly, orderly, and effectively, and the dilemma continues. The deficit in communication skills only exacerbates the dilemma and invariably reflects on the pay scale of the worker.

As our population ages, people living longer, it is projected that health care workers will be among the fastest-growing job opportunities in the next decade. This, however, is not the only reason for difficulties in finding trained, motivated, and dedicated workers; equally important are the conditions of work, the nature of work, and the inequity in compensation of health care workers. It is quickly forgotten that a chain is as strong as its weakest link. The average care worker earning $10 an *hour*, varying from state to state, has to work at least two jobs in order to earn a livable wage, just above or at the poverty level. Many believe that the solution will not be resolved merely by pumping money into the system. The solution more relates to the elimination of the vast waste and excessive compensations which are pervasive throughout the health care system and a more transparent and equitable distribution of the funds already allocated to the system. It is paradoxical that the most ardent critics of the system happen to be recipients of the largest largess. Other links in the chain are the physicians/specialists, registered nurses (RN), licensed practical nurses (LPN), and secretarial staff; these individuals play an important role in keeping the chain intact.

The Attending Physicians: The role of the physician is clear. It is an important and indispensable one. Every patient admitted to an acute care, subacute care, or extended care facility must have medical clearance and assigned to a physician who would be the primary care physician during the stay in the institution. Some facility may accept clearance by the family physician. Attending physicians, who are privileged to care for clients, are credentialed by the institution before being admitted to the staff. These physicians are not usually employed by the institution. They see patients on a fee-for-service arrangement. Your primary care physician is able to seek consultations by specialists usually in consultation with patients or family members. There is no obligation to retain these physicians, but whoever is selected must be licensed by state and credentialed by the institution. Physicians will usually bill Medicare for the service rendered. Medicare may pay up to 80 percent of the amount it approved; the patient or his insurers pay the 20 percent.

I have had complaints from patients and their family members that family physicians were not permitted to care for their medical needs while in skilled nursing facility (SNF). They complained of having to go through a litany of medical tests and procedures which were recently done and well known to the family physician.

"Why should I give up my right to my own doctor for one who may be less experienced and competent or one who has difficulty understanding me?" (communication). These complaints are not uncommon and not without merits; my suspicion is, they will increase as skilled facilities and other institutions struggle in recruiting experienced physicians to fill these openings. Many U.S.-trained physicians are reluctant to serve these facilities. My experience as one who was involved in recruitment of new physicians has shown that for every one experienced U.S.-trained physician applicant, there were four applicants who were graduates from foreign medical schools. Since all candidates presented identical post-graduate medical certifications, it was assumed that they all have met the same requirements for patient care. I have also monitored some U.S. medical graduates whose services I would not recommend. All foreign graduates need not be painted with one broad brush regarding their medical and communication skills. Physicians with whom I have spoken, complained about the very low salary paid by institutions to house physicians who do have considerable responsibilities as one reason for the inability to recruit more highly trained and experienced physicians. Some physicians are attracted to institutional employment because of difficulties in competing for positions at the highly rated university-affiliated centers. They are more likely to be accepted at the peripheral hospitals, some with university affiliation.

To have your family physician caring for your medical needs in a skilled nursing facility is not always an easy task. All institutions have standards for admission to their medical staff. Except for some state county and municipal institutions, the admission to a hospital staff is very restrictive and sometimes exclusionary. In days of yore, black physician applicants were summarily disqualified for being black. The process is less racially influenced today, but barriers still exist. Many graduates of foreign medical schools are also excluded from certain institutions. In addition to having your office and practice within the catchment area of the institution, there must be a need for your specialty at the institution. Then there is the question of qualifications.

Preference is usually given to U.S. medical graduates at many institutions. Whether a candidate is certified by a specialty board or merely eligible, may be another criterion. The number of specialists in a given specialty is another deciding factor. If a community hospital had an overwhelming number of orthopedists on its attending staff, there may be reluctance to admit another orthopedist to the attending staff; it then becomes a <u>case</u> of protection of one's turf. Some applicants have had to take their case to court. Physicians covering SNF should be ever mindful of their exclusive dominance, more often without the will of the patients, and go out of their way to be courteous and professional in their relationship with clients and family members; they should never take advantage of their exclusive status. A patient's right to choose his/her doctor is still paramount, more so with the Affordable Care Act.

The RN and LPN: These are members of the ward staff and are responsible for carrying out orders prescribed by the attending physician caring for the patients. All registered nurses and licensed practical nurses must be certified by the state. They must also be credentialed by the institution and registered to practice their profession within the state. The difference between the RN and LPN is a narrow one and differs in respect of length of training, the periods for the RN being longer than for the LPN. The registered nurse usually carries out the initial assessment of new patients and issues certain certifying documents. To conserve operating cost and satisfy state requirements, many skilled nursing care facilities have employed licensed practical nurses (LPN) to fulfill certain functions of the RN. Registered nurses (RN) at many facilities are preoccupied, sometimes overwhelmed, by paperwork or computerized documentation to ensure that all procedures which relate to patient care are recorded. They take physicians' orders by telephone; they ensure that patients' appointments for clinics and activities are kept; they communicate certain information to family or advocates of patients. They evaluate and certify patients for transfer from one institution to another. A number of these functions could only be carried out by the RN. I have seen RNs so fixed on documentation that an eye contact with a family member standing in front of them is a precious and time-consuming commodity which they can ill afford. I am told that the reason for such intense documentation has to do with requirements for state accreditation.

This dichotomy of functions of the RN and LPN has led to misinformation when I inquired about the vital signs of my patient who had developed lethargy and increased heart rate. Because of the prior history, I had suspected urinary tract infection. I was told by the RN that the vital signs of my patient were all normal. Not fully satisfied with this report, I asked the LPN and was told that the vital signs of my patient were abnormal. In addition, she was running a fever. This contradictory information was given a few minutes apart. As it transpired, the LPN was correct.

In another case, I inquired from the RN whether my patient had received his medication. She was unable to give any information on such a fundamentally important question and suggested that I ask the LPN. There seem to be a developing new trend in nursing where skilled nursing is no longer carried out by registered nurses (RNs) but by licensed practical nurses (LPNs) and the caregivers. Higher degrees in nursing are desirable, but this further removes the RN from the patients and from nursing as we know it. They have become clerks. As a clinical clerk at a regional hospital in the United Kingdom, ward rounds were looked upon as a unique and teaching experience; it was more than a casual encounter with patients. Our ward rounds were led by the ward sister and the consulting physician, then the senior house officer, followed by the lesser rank. Every medical patient was seen and discussed. The ward sister virtually leads the team, updating the consultant and the senior house officer on current status of each patient in textbook fashion. There was no need to consult an LPN; they had none. At the end of the session, we assembled at the nursing office for discussions about special needs of patients and any related problems. Then of course, tea was served.

Ward rounds in New York were quite different. No nurses were present, the resident presented his case, and of course, there was no tea, a great disappointment. I wondered, how could a ward round be terminated without a cup of tea?

THE PHYSIATRIST AND PHYSICAL REHABILITATION

PHYSIATRIST: The terms physiatrist and physiatry were introduced in 1938 by the late Frank H. Krusen. It was adapted by the American Medical Association in 1946 and became more universally accepted following World War II, when injured soldiers returned from the war.

The physiatrist as leader of the Physical Rehabilitation team: When one thinks of Physical Rehabilitation of a stroke patient, also those with muscle/skeletal diseases and with problems entirely related to the aging process, the physiatrist has been active. In most centers, the rehabilitation specialist, the physiatrist, heads the management team. He/She is a physician who has a medical degree, often with other specialized training, and certifications such as neurology, orthopedics, and internal medicine. He/She has studied the disease pathways and functions of the various systems and able to evaluate, analyze, and prescribe definitive treatments for problems affecting these systems. As a certified specialist, he/she is often able to predict the course of the progress and give evidence as an expert witness in a court of law. The physiatrist treats a wide range of conditions, including arthritis; stroke; musculoskeletal pain syndromes, such as low back pain, rehabilitation in cardiopulmonary disease; fibromyalgia; traumatic brain injury. The goal is to enable the individual achieve maximum functions within the limits of his/her capacity and to enhance the quality of life.

It is believed that about 250,000 people will seek some form of physical rehabilitation management after a stroke; this is in addition to the present number of people with other neuromuscular and locomotion problems. The department of physical medicine and rehabilitation (PM&R) in virtually every large medical center in the United States is chaired by a specialist in Rehabilitation Medicine. In the normal course of events, stroke patients are routinely referred to the department of PM&R for evaluation and management. These patients are examined by a physiatrist or resident physician, their functional status is determined and accordingly, a definitive rehabilitation program is constructed. It is usual to include physical therapy, occupational therapy, speech/hearing therapy after these evaluations. It is a common misconception to assume that a prescription for physical therapy and occupational therapy represent a prescription for therapy. These orders in my view, merely call the attention of the physical therapist and the occupational therapist to these new patients A definitive prescription should be written after evaluation which corresponds to the patient's need.

For the stroke patient with weakness, a definitive prescription may be written for:

1. Physical Therapy including General conditioning exercises, active and active-assistive range of motion, progressing to Progressive Resistive exercise

2. Trunk strengthening exercises, progressing to independent sitting.

3. Standing, balancing progressing to gait training; progress to walker, cane, stairs and independence.

Occupational therapy for: General conditioning and Activities of Daily Living (ADL) Note: There is a progression in the series of exercises for physical therapy. It is assumed that if the patient has generalized weakness to the extent that he/she is unable to sit, it is unlikely that he would be expected to stand or walk.

Knowing the medical history of your patient and with your own medical background, you, the physiatrist, are in the best position to offer caution to the physical therapist or occupational therapist relative to the limits of therapy on individual patient. This important responsibility should not be left entirely to the whims of the therapists. Most therapists welcome this insightful collaboration with the referring physician. It often serves as a unique learning experience for both.

Too often, physicians abdicate their responsibilities to the physiotherapist and the occupational therapist to the extent that they are no longer able or willing to write a definitive prescription for specific muscles, joints, or functions; these should always be foremost when prescribing. I have seen prescription written for "ambulation exercise." This is the same as prescribing "walk the patient." It should not require a medical degree and a specialist certification to prescribe ambulate or walk a patient who otherwise has no medical contraindication. If the prescriber had written a caution, that may have given some validity to the prescription. Needless to say, billing for this absurdity is rejected by Medicare and Medicaid when presented for payment.

Another frequent omission, physiatrists do not observe their patients in the rehabilitation environment (therapy areas) to see how they function. There is an overreliance on the PT and OT reports without verification. This omission poses great risk in certifying functional improvement or decline when in fact the opposite is in operation. What if your patient is malingering? However, physical therapists, as important members of the physical rehabilitation team, cannot be overemphasized; the role of the physiatrist as leader of the team is not minimized.

I have long felt that management of the stroke patient should be a team approach; the patient is best served when this is an integrated management. The key players are the internist, the neurologist, and the physiatrist. The internist is usually the personal or attending physician and is familiar with the patient's health and will most likely be responsible for the ongoing management of the patient, including problems which may have precipitated the stroke. Some of these problems may have been some of the risk factors mentioned earlier in this book. The family physician, the internist, is likely to have been the first to make the diagnosis then consulted other members of the management team.

PHYSIATRIST: After the patient is evaluated by a neurologist, who makes a definitive diagnosis, various tests and procedures may be carried out to confirm the diagnosis, and the patient may be admitted. The neurologist may continue to monitor and treat until the patient is stabilized. The internist or the neurologist may then request the consultation of the physiatrist who will evaluate the patient and determine the extent of the patient's disability and then conceptualize a comprehensive physical rehabilitation program for the course of the hospital stay and beyond. The rehabilitation team may include physical therapist, occupational therapist, speech and hearing therapist, and social services.

For many stroke patients, some form of physical rehabilitation program should become an ongoing course if optimum health care is to be achieved. There is the tendency for stroke patients to develop contractures which limit movement in joints of the affected extremities. Immobility also causes restrictions in other joints and body movements. The program indicated for this group is not the heroic body building exercise program. Wheelchair clients/patients with potentials should be encouraged to propel their chairs using the lower extremities. Alternate forward and backward bending, the rocking chair exercise is also beneficial for the immobilized clients/patients; it promotes movements for the trunk and extremities and increases the circulation and function of the heart. Correction of faulty and inappropriate posture should receive attention. Wheel-chaired patients unable to make these corrections should receive the ongoing attention of trained members of the staff. As simple as these procedures may appear, they should only be done with the sanction and approval of the registered physical therapy staff, who is more familiar with the body mechanics, and the attending physician, who is familiar with the medical contraindications of his patients.

When a patient with an old CVA and left-sided weakness was admitted through the emergency room in a nonresponsive, semiconscious state with flaccidity and hyporeflexia, several CT scans were negative for new damage to the brain (infarcts). Electrolytes were abnormal with potassium as low as two, the EKG showing S-T segment depression and inverted T waves. There were also frequent muscle spasms and contractions over the cheek and chest. A diagnosis of CVA and seizure disorder was entertained. The dissenting view came from the physiatrist who stated his diagnosis as electrolytes disorder with severe hypopotassemia. The patient showed remarkable changes and verbalized, following restoration of electrolytes balance. It transpired that patient was on diuretic without potassium supplement for months. A learning experience.

I am yet to see a new or old stroke admitted in a virtual comatose/semi-comatose state, flaccidity and hyporeflexia in extremities, who has responded so dramatically to restoration of electrolytes and with no new focal weakness. However, I have examined many senior patients admitted with the diagnosis of CVA who miraculously recovered overnight after restoration of electrolytes balance, an interesting learning experience for interns and residents.

THE PHYSIATRIST: It was helpful that the physiatrist, because of his medical background, was able to correlate the patient's history with the laboratory and EKG findings and formed an independent impression which correlated with the final diagnosis. The patient suffered no new weakness. It follows, therefore, that physiatrists, although seeking the opinion of other specialists, must themselves analyze all supporting data available and at least have a tentative diagnostic impression. At the same time, the role of the physical therapist and occupational therapist should not be minimized. They are important links in the chain. However, it is the role of the physiatrist to exercise his/her medical judgment by offering restrictions to any therapeutic modalities which in their view may result in harm to the patient. They should also be able to prescribe medications which may facilitate the outcome of therapy carried out by the physical therapist.

A common error in physical rehabilitation (PT/OT) management is the failure to extend their influences beyond the narrow limits of the therapy areas. This is especially true in the subacute rehabilitation facility where the goal seems to be meeting the mandatory minimum time requirement of three hours of therapy tolerance each day. The patient/client is then cared for by the nurses (RN/LPN), aides, companion, many of whom have no knowledge about the therapy objectives. Some centers have trained rehabilitation nurses who continue to guide the course of rehabilitation and provide some carryover of therapy. Most of those admitted for acute or subacute physical rehabilitation also present with significant medical problems which also have to be addressed.

COMMON DEFORMITIES: Typical deformities of many stroke and some bed-bound patients are flexion, adduction, and internal rotation. In the upper extremity, adduction and flexion at the shoulder, elbow, wrist, and digits of the hands; the extremity is rotated inward. Similarly, the lower extremities tend to adduct and rotate inward with flexion at the hip and knee. The neck and shoulder for the most part are in flexion, largely from faulty posturing. With these expected structural changes, physical rehabilitation should have some carryover, extending to the patient's living and sleeping arrangements.

Most patients spend about three or four hours daily in physical therapy. The next twenty hours are often spent undoing some of the functions gained during the course of their rehabilitation intervention, unwittingly. All support services (nurses and aides) should have at least some idea of the therapy objective of patients they serve. This is the essence of the chain approach to physical rehabilitation. All members of the chain are important.

I have seen patients discharged from hospital and rehabilitation facilities with deformities which were not present at the time of admission, an embarrassment for any institution. This is tantamount to iatrogenic medicine where the result from therapy was worse. I have also seen a patient whose cervical flexion deformity was so severe that she was unable to look at her favorite television programs. Muscle relaxant taken by mouth and by topical infiltration were said to have been only minimally effective.

Cervical deformities noted were the result of patient sleeping in her chair, day and night instead of sleeping in her bed. The patient who lived alone and had maintained mobility but began sleeping in a chair because she was unable to get in and out of her bed because of severe arthritic pain during the process of bed transfer. She had converted her bed to a desk using a wide board to support her writing paper. After several months, she developed severe flexion of her neck, so she was unable to raise her head to look at the television. The patient was admitted for subacute rehabilitation. Within two weeks of her admission, she was able to look at her television programs sitting erectly in her chair.

The miraculous resolution to her problem came about with little structured physical rehabilitation intervention but with the intervention of nursing staff and the patient. The cause of her problem was carefully explained, and the therapy required to cure her problem was also explained. Only one soft pillow was provided for sleeping and a roll under the small of her neck; there was also some support for the upper trunk.

After the first week of postural positioning, the change was dramatic. The patient had virtually taken over her therapy after she experienced the dramatic changes. Simply put, gravity had resolved what gravity had initiated. Her neck was in extension during sleep merely by positioning.

POSITIONING: Positioning of patients, especially in the skilled nursing facility (SNF), deserves special attention. It is an area often overlooked by nurses and caregivers; attending physicians concentrate on prescribing medications; administrators are too far removed. My interest was drawn to this simple but important aspect of patient care after observing the crippling effect of faulty positioning of patients both in their homes and in nursing facilities.

Senior patients, often with evidence of dementia, are placed in wheelchairs or standard chairs during the day; they receive no structured physical therapy or physical exercises; many are on medications, including antiseizure medications, which induce somnolence (sleep). Their heads and necks are continually in flexion. This experience is readily verified by entering any dayroom or other sitting areas, even in the best SNF. There is no doubt that some of the somnolence-induced neck flexion is the direct effect of medications. Physicians are timid to readjust these highly sedating medications, some for seizure disorder, because they doggedly follow the advice of their local pharmacist or the representatives (reps) of the pharmaceutical companies who are adept in selling drugs but have little insight in the care of patients. Some physicians are afraid to reduce the "therapeutic dose" recommended by the drug manufacturers; they fail to take into account variables which influence the action of the medications they prescribe, even though the patients sleep their lives away and develop deformities in the process.

The sequence should continue with trunk-strengthening exercises and sitting balance, postural exercises, bed mobility, active and active-assistive range of motion with gentle stretching in the cervical, upper extremities, and lower extremities. The rationale for stretching is to counter the tendency for flexion, adduction, and internal rotation common in the stroke patient. The application of heat or cold prior to ranging is sometimes helpful in relaxing tight muscles and joints. A series of progressive-resistive exercises should be implemented to strengthen the muscles of the extremities and trunk. The physiotherapist/occupational therapist often use their expertise to formulate and carry out the appropriate programs. Eventual gait training to facilitate independent ambulation or ambulation with assistive device, with the aid of the parallel bars and mirror, these are essential to facilitate self-correction and reciprocal gait. Braces or splints when indicated, especially brace for dorsiflexion assist, plays a very important role; assist in ankle dorsiflexion tends to limit circumduction at the hip and facilitates gait training.

Flexion Deformity in the Neck: I have devoted time to this problem because of its frequent occurrence in seniors and post-stroke patients. I have observed similar changes in wheelchair-bound patients in nursing homes. My interest has led me to examine the cervical (neck) x-ray of seniors sixty-five and over; I also examined cervical skeletons. I found in many a reduction in height of the body of each bone in the neck (vertebrae) which I describe as wedged shape; the base of the wedge is posterior, and the apex is anterior or ventral. I hasten to add that these findings are not new but well established. These changes may determine the curve in the neck as we age. Any condition or posture which exacerbates these structural changes will influence the curve in the neck. In the stroke patient, flexion of the neck is exacerbated by contracture of muscles; two muscles commonly involved in forward flexion are the sternomastoid and portion of the trapezius. When the sternomastoid contracts, the neck bends forward or to one side. In time and without therapy, these deformities may become fixed. Treatment may then require relaxant medication, splinting, even surgical intervention. This deformity may be prevented or significantly delayed with appropriate posturing. This is a much neglected modality in skilled nursing facilities (SNF) where the specialty of physiatry is unknown. It is regrettable that positioning as a preventive or delaying measure against cervical deformities, especially in the stroke patient, is hardly undertaken. Rehabilitation nursing is virtually nonexistent, and there seem to be little or no understanding of simple body mechanics. Many patients are positioned in bed or in chair in positions which only hasten the onset of crippling deformities.

MEDICAL CARE: Many of the medical problems experienced by seniors and others confined to assisted or skilled nursing facilities are adequately addressed by physicians assigned to these facilities and, when feasible, by their personal physicians. Many of these physicians have training in internal medicine. Some physicians have specialized training in elder care or geriatric medicine; they are generally dedicated and well able to cope with the usual medical emergencies. When events occur beyond their reach, consultants and/or hospital referrals are generally available so that the medical/surgical needs of residents are fully met. There are, however, exceptions especially in smaller facilities where there are reports of long delays to access the services of physicians and much reliance is placed on the registered nurse (RN) in charge.

It can be argued that, in spite of these problems, the care at most institutions is preferred to having seniors remain in their homes with less support services. However, I have found significant neglect of the physical/functional and locomotion needs of many wheel-chaired residents. I reject the notion that clients/patients confined to wheelchairs cannot benefit from functional activities; this notion, unfortunately, seems to have purveyed the thinking of many administrators and caregivers involved in care, including victims of arthritis, muscular diseases, stroke, or just the inevitable process of ageing. Such thinking is the antithesis to reality as many professionals in physical rehabilitation have observed. This philosophy must be changed if those confined to institutions and wheelchairs are to receive full and equal attention and benefits.

Some wheel-chaired patients in SNF are involved in some of the social programs available, but these are limited to bingo and musical activities for small groups. Although these social events are necessary, they do not fill the need for motor activities. This void in physical activities is due to the perception by administrators and caregivers that wheelchair—and bed-bound patients do not require motor stimulation. There is the erroneous belief that only those who are able to walk or can participate in other modalities will benefit from exercise programs. To refute these perceptions, reference is made of a distinguished professor and chairman of a department, who told me "The daily exercise program for my upper body has kept me in shape for years." This distinguished physician had been injured during the war and was paralyzed in the lower extremities; he functioned as paraplegic from his wheelchair, and for all practical purposes, he lived a full and independent life. He was not unique; there are many such citizens, including veterans, who are wheelchair-bound and fully employed but also benefit from motion exercises to preserve and enhance those functions which require body movements. In the real world, we do not neglect the medical needs of our patients because their mental functions are compromised; they continue to receive their blood pressure medications and their blood sugar medications. Conversely, we should not neglect other functional needs of patients whose ability to walk are compromised and are relegated to wheelchair status. The practice by some institutions of offering custody while charging for skilled care, irrespective of the per diem cost, is not uncommon and should be addressed. It is not uncommon to see wheel-chaired patients slumped in their chairs with arm dangling over the side armrest of the chair, both legs suspended in air with incredible stress to the hip joint and lower back. These occurrences are within the full view of nurses and aides sitting comfortably at their station and ignoring the postural strain being imposed on their charges in wheelchair. Correction of this simple position neglect did not require an advanced degree in physical therapy to recognize and to address. The knee-jerk denial will be quickly applied when this neglect is brought to the attention of any supervisor. Hence, no correction is effected, and patients suffer needlessly. I have expressed amazement that with such prolonged and abnormal posture, more patients do not develop the brachial plexus palsy, also referred to as the Saturday night palsy or the armchair palsy. This paralysis, often transient in nature, is due to stretching of the brachial plexus as it traverses through the axilla (armpit). Most victims make full recovery in time once the cause of the stretch is resolved. The lesson to be learned is that this condition may be prevented with correct positioning. Any layman can correct the position of a patient slumped in a wheelchair if it is recognized that the position is harmful to the client/patient and there is the will to do something positive.

What was lacking in many instances are basic common sense, understanding the principles of positioning of wheelchair patients, and the will to execute. This was especially true of stroke patients in wheelchair. There must be some basic in-service training for care workers, not on paper for the inspectors but in practice. There must also be responsible, respectable, and capable supervisors who can command the respect of those workers under her/his charge. I concede that with ratio of staff to patient of one to ten and one to twelve, even a simple postural correction may be an imposition into the time of a care worker. It is well established that crippling deformities do occur in skilled nursing facilities; these can be reduced by attending to the simple problem of positioning, especially of the wheel-chaired patients and those confined to bed.

CHALLENGING PROBLEMS: Challenging rehabilitation problems to the health care system are those obscured conditions to which seniors are most susceptible and which I have previously reported (*Geriatrics Journal*) I refer to the syndrome of: " Central Cervical Cord Compression". This syndrome has been well researched and published by others in rehabilitation and other specialties. It is well known that trauma is the primary cause, but preexisting degenerative changes found, especially in the elderly, render them more susceptible to this unique injury and distribution of weakness. This syndrome in younger patients is frequently *associated* with compression fracture or fracture-dislocation of the cervical vertebra, the result of automobile accident or diving injuries.

In contrast to the classical quadriplegia (weakness in four extremities), in paralysis of the central cord, the lower extremities are less involved, and the impairment of function is more severe in the upper extremities. There is invariably bladder and bowel incontinent; these patients also show a characteristic pattern of recovery with initial return of motor function in the lower extremities followed by improvement of bladder and bowel function; eventually, there is varying degree of recovery in the upper extremities. Improvement in the intrinsic muscles of the hand is variable and protracted.

In injuries to the spine, it is important that the attending physicians distinguish between those cases where early operative intervention is indicated and those that require conservative management, including an extended program of physical rehabilitation. The management of cervical spine injuries with cord involvement remains controversial. Some specialists (R.C. Schneider

J. Neuro. Surg.) believe that early operative intervention is indicated when there is

- Immediate complete paralysis with diminished sensation at a certain level
- Progression of the neurologic signs
- Fracture of spine associated with leak of spinal fluids
- Marked encroachment of bony fragments upon spinal canal
- Evidence of a complete block of spinal fluid on jugular compression

TRAINING: Physical rehabilitation for seniors/disabled should continue in some measure in their home environment if the problem of recidivism with hospital/rehabilitation admissions is to be controlled. This may require some oversight to check their functional status and provide timely intervention when needed. Such oversight may be carried out by the home caregiver who is given orientation in some of the early signs of problems, such as recognition of skin abrasions and blisters, recognition of tightness and pain in joints during their care.

One staff nurse (LPN) could not distinguish a fulminant skin rash from "goose pimples" to alert the attending physician. She neglected to alert the attending physician when asked to do so by the patient's advocate, a licensed physician.

The case referenced in this publication of a patient who was admitted with deformities in the neck; this should have been discovered early by the home care aides, reported and corrected in the home. This observation by the home care worker would have prevented a hospital admission or an emergency room visit; this home care dilemma would have been resolved. The home care workers are often the sole guardian of many seniors who live at home. However, many lack the experience or judgment to recognize some of the simple indicators of serious structural problems. The training needed for these workers need not be prodigious or complicated. A practical in-service or on-the-job demonstration may be adequate for some workers who have already acquired certain basic skills. Workers with language impediment may be less suitable for this training. Alternatively, the visiting nurse who already has many basic skills may be suitably adapted to cover this task.

A word of caution, in several facilities I visited, the structural design and some amenities seem to be conceptualized mainly to enhance the ambience of the surrounding room or apartment with disregard for the functional ability of the clients served. Two common impediments have come to my attention: handrails and floor covering. In one facility, the handrail along the wall was a beautifully polished rectangular-shaped wooden strip which was carefully designed and coordinated with the color of the wall in the background. This was thought to be very attractive, and it was to the designer/architect and administrators who apparently were ignorant of the rehabilitation objectives. It was a veritable disaster for the handicapped whose flexors of the hand were so weak that a built-up rounded-handle spoon was necessary to enhance ability to self-feed. This was in fact an impediment to client's effort to rehabilitate and restore functional grasp. He/she was never able to grasp this rectangular rail and could not practice independent ambulation in the room, stairs, or hallway. This emphasizes the need for cooperation between designers and specialists in rehabilitation.

PHYSICAL REHABILITATION:

The other impediments are the loosely scattered rugs on the floor which in my judgment only serve as hazardous trapping which function is to create a dangerous environment for the physically compromised individual who invariably is also troubled by visual deficits. This problem is easily resolved by donating these trappings to family, friends, the Salvation Army, or similar charitable organizations. The big offender seems to be the wall-to-wall carpet covering the floor space.

During my early years in practice, I was asked by a friend to see one of his patients, also his friend who was just recovering from a stroke, in consultation. This seventy-four-year-old gentleman had suffered a stroke about a year previously and had resumed his usual work as an executive. His chief complaint was increasing tiredness and fatigue in his legs. His difficulty was worse walking at home at the end of the day. His physician recommended less walking at work, believing that the problem was related to stress at work; but his job was in fact sedentary. To do less walking would have meant taking a cot to work and lying during the day, a perfect example for his work crew. In addition to his diagnosis of a stroke, he was troubled by degenerative arthritis, which was diagnosed incidentally because he had no overt symptoms.

My limited examination found left hemiparesis with functional range. Muscle strength ranged from 3+/5 distally and 4/5 proximally. My question was why was he tired and fatigued after work when his work was sedentary and required virtually no walking? After walking through his family room, then upstairs, and walking through his living room to his study on the upper floor, the diagnosis was very apparent because the consulting physician was himself becoming tired and fatigued in both lower extremities. This gentleman had what was then known and fashionable as "shaggy rug" throughout his split-level home. With relative weakness in his hip flexors, quads, and ankle dorsiflexors, his effort to retrieve his left lower extremity from this thick rug with the resistance it imposed, exacerbated his weakness and induced his fatigue. It was one of the quickest and easiest diagnoses in my medical career. The problem was in his wall-to-wall shaggy rug. Yet some facilities insist on the installation of thick heavy floor covering because this enhances the ambience of the rooms or apartments. They ignore the fact that occupants should be able to function (walking) in their homes. They seem to rely on the opinion of the interior decorator for this decision-making process.

It was a learning experience, not from the textbook but from practice. Wall-to-wall carpeting should offer only minimum resistance to ambulation or wheelchair propulsion. The physically challenged welcomes and appreciates the beauty of the environment but one where they are also able to function and improve their residual capacities to the maximum. A thick wall-to-wall carpet or scattered floor rugs are not the appropriate environment.

Senior Care

ADD ONE MORE PILL: The abundance of pills we prescribe for senior citizens has gotten out of control, and this was reinforced by my personal experience. A senior citizen who was admitted to three institutions within a period of six months and left each institution with at least one additional prescription,to the long list of medications she was already prescribed. Does a patient need a pill for every symptom or perceived symptom reported? I reject the notion that the physician must prescribe a tablet, capsule, elixir, or injection for every sign or symptom presented by his patient. This practice only resulted in another set of medications for the medicine cabinet.

Physicians and medical personnel are under teremendous pressure, coping with the increasing number of patients who invade emergency rooms and hospitals. Many of the signs and symptoms described by some patients are the result of anxiety emanating from stress and strains of daily living. In earlier years, these signs were manifested mainly by senior citizens. Today younger patients are seen in emergency rooms with similar problems; they are real to the patient and should be carefully and professionally addressed. There should be no place for a dismissive attitude on the part of the physicians, for the one you dismiss may be the professional decision you live to regret. However, adding one more pill may impose unnecessary burden on your patient, especially seniors who will carry this to the next institution. This scenario repeats itself from institution to institution, and the senior becomes the inevitable pharmacy. Fortunately, many patients show better judgment than the prescriber, and those pills hastily prescribed become collector's items in the patients' medicine cabinets. This may be dismissed as a laughable encounter, but the dilemma we confront is why and who pays for such unnecessary extravagance.

Physicians are expected to treat their patients, but treat what? One senior was very impressed that her doctor had given her the best treatment she had received in years. Her physician simply palpated her abdomen, percussed her chest, listened to her heart, and took her pressure. He then took her knee and ankle reflexes and had her walk. Her only problem was constipation, which he assured her was common with people who do not exercise and whose diets have changed. He suggested more roughage in her diet. What she perceived as treatment was simply a routine physical examination.

I have heard others bitterly complaining, "I spent two hours in this office, and would you believe, he didn't even give me a prescription after the examination?" Many people have come to expect something, at least a prescription, after being examined by their physician. There is no doubt patients have also contributed to this habit of writing another prescription after examination. The art of a good physical examination proved to be therapeutic. My Scottish consultant has always reminded his house staff, "Don't neglect to take the pulse. It is your bread and butter in medical practice."

Why are seniors stuck with one more pill? Because it is easier and more convenient to maintain the status quo. In order to alter a previously prescribed medication, the physician must reexamine the patient, review the supporting laboratory and clinical reports, and review the patient's history. This is a time-consuming process for many physicians who are perhaps already burdened by a heavy and disproportionate patient load. Perhaps the most compelling reason is the fear of making the wrong decision. One way to justify the status quo is to leave it alone. "I did not prescribe the medication. The prescribing physician will have to alter or discontinue its use." The underlying fear of being sued if things go wrong is also a real dilemma. This scenario leaves the patient with a needless medication, which may harm him/her, and does nothing to alleviate the present problems, yet another set of pills for the medicine cabinet.

There is reason to believe that the pillars of health care delivery are the care workers/aides, those who at 6:00 a.m., 7:00, a.m., 8:00 a.m., *and* beyond are on the job to carry out the daily routine. They empty the urinals, toilet their clients/patients, participate in their cleaning-up (showers, oral hygiene and/or bed baths). They dress and feed those requiring assistance and have them prepared and ready for doctor's appointments and other scheduled activities for the day. Although training for the tasks they perform required less time than that required for nurses and other support staff, to function as they do must require a unique capacity and dedication which are often taken for granted. They undoubtedly must have some love for the sick and disabled, a level of physical and mental fortitude and ingenuity to survive on the marginal income they receive for their service.

Who are these men and women of the health care pyramid? They are the workers who live at or below the poverty level and among the "47 percent," though they work one or two full-time jobs. Many of these workers are recent immigrants or immigrants residing in the United States for several years. They are the pillars which sustain the health care system. I have doubt that the system will collapse in the absence of top-level administrators. However, I have seen chaos and disruption of basic services when care workers are unexpectedly absent; a chain of events occurred, including changes in doctor's scheduled appointments, clients not being fed in a timely manner, clients remained soiled for excessively long periods; these changes would hardly have occurred if the CEO or other high level administrators were absent or never appeared for work. It should also be remembered that complaints about the quality of care never relate to the administrative staff. Many victims of abuse are seldom aware of the existence of a CEO or president.

In spite of all the good intent, care workers may carry out some tasks in manner which fail to benefit their clients/patients but solely for the benefit of the care worker. This is done to the detriment of the clients/patients. One aide who persistently used the basin provided for patient's personal sanitary needs as the receptacle for the patient's oral care. She refused to use the "kidney basin" specially designed and provided for that purpose. She loudly protested when asked to use the "kidney basin" for oral hygiene. Her claim being that the kidney basin was too small, and it was easier for her to manage with the large sanitary basin. There was a total disconnect between the rehabilitation objectives and the care provided by the aide. Her client will be using a "kidney basin" for oral hygiene upon her discharge but had no practice using this device in rehabilitation. There was also a disregard for basic sanitary principles. I have observed, with dismay, caregiver/aide placing the patient's toothbrush in the very sink where she had just emptied the waste water after morning wash-up of her client/patient. The toothbrush was discarded on my insistence. In all these undertakings, the aide dutifully kept on her gloves. Everything within her reach was then well contaminated with soiled gloves. Hand washing was not a priority with the false notion that by wearing the same pair of gloves for all activities, there would be absolute protection. It is fortunate that the body offers natural resistance to many contaminant bacteria. I hasten to mention that these infractions on the part of care workers are not vindictive or malicious but sadly reflect an environment and health codes which differ from those generally accepted in the United States. The larger question is where are the supervisors, and what level of training did these workers experience?

TRAINING: Many care workers have little or no structured training in caring for the elderly and disabled; their expectation is "on-the-job training." Many of them present certificates indicating licenses or registration, although verbal communication was at its lowest level and some care workers are incapable of documenting the work covered during their tour of duty. There are many home care training centers competing for potential health care workers. It is said that the need for trained health care workers has outpaced the available centers for training these candidates. This dilemma undoubtedly pressures agencies and institutions competing for the limited number of trained personnel to an extent that they may register anyone claiming experience or training as a health care worker/aide. Some care workers have high school certificate, many with GED certificates. However, many of the immigrants and recent immigrant workers are without any documentation of school certification. It is often very difficult to evaluate the academic standing of these workers due to varying educational standards and language barriers. Many of these workers are without creditable academic certification; in fact, some may be barely literate in the country of origin. Fortunately, little direct documentation of their work activities is necessary; these are usually reported to the RN or LPN in charge of the unit. This deficiency does not negate nor minimize the outstanding contributions of many immigrant workers to the health care delivery system. In many institutions, the immigrant workers represent the largest contingent of health care workers charged with the responsibility of the care of residents. This workforce includes directors and supervising staff and those responsible for housekeeping.

CRITERIA EVALUATED: Younger workers impart a sense of haste in attending the needs of the seniors. They are said to be more likely to work by the clock, on occasions leaving the client partially clothed to be attended by the relieving staff. Older workers showed more empathy and patience, somewhat slower but more thorough in their work. The exceptional young worker, however, has debunked this notion.

Ethnicity: There was the perception that minority workers, especially from the Caribbean, were more caring of the elderly; they showed greater empathy and patience in attending to the needs of their clients. Other care workers were perceived to show a disconnect with seniors in general and with minorities in particular. My experience contradicts this perception that workers from the Caribbean showed greater empathy and care for their clients.

EYE CONTACT: Although this mode of assessment is well known and has been used frequently in psychological evaluation, I underestimated its importance as a tool to determine the candor and reliability of information obtained in the course of an interview. I caution, however, that there can be erroneous conclusion drawn from eye contact; ethnicity, culture, sex may play a role. However, I found interesting correlation with eye contact and reliability of information given by home care workers. Although the nature of infractions was not critical, their cumulative effect could have resulted in increased morbidity of clients/patients. One should only apply this entity with due consideration of factor mentioned, always giving the benefit of doubt to the care worker. I have applied this theory to a number of care workers, including professionals, with some success.

My experience with eye contact has left an indelible imprint on me. I have used this with others modalities to develop the "Quality Care Assessment Scale" to group standings of health care facilities. I relate my own experience mentioned in my book *A Successful Journey, Not Without Pain*. I applied for a vacant position at a large teaching hospital on the recommendation of an attending physician at the same hospital. I was given an appointment for an interview by the chief of service of the department. I was very prompt for the interview, arriving there about 8:30 a.m. for my 9:00 a.m. interview. When I arrived, the secretary announced my arrival to the chief and ushered me to his office. When I entered, he was sitting in a swing chair behind his desk. He raised his head as I entered the office, long enough to recognize me but with absolutely no further eye contact. It was an amusing encounter; but I was not amused. He immediately swung the chair around facing the wall and a credenza, or book case, with his back facing me as I stood there sweating profusely in the palm of my hands and in total disbelief of what was happening. As he fiddled with papers in his hands, still facing the credenza he said to me: "Sorry you had to travel all that distance; we have no position open; we did not receive the grants we expected to cover salaries." Still no eye contact. He then stood up, meaning the end of the interview and in this situation it implied to me: "You get the hell out of my office. Throughout this ordeal I was never offered a seat or eye contact. He did express regret for my useless travel. It was a humiliating experience that still haunts me. It was interesting to note that the position was advertised for weeks after this despicable encounter. I was told later that he was still interviewing candidates for the position for which no grants were received to cover salaries. The avoidance of eye contact was quite telling of his character, he was not truthful.

DURATION OF EMPLOYMENT: Where workers had been in continuous employment for a short period, less than 5 years, the quality of care was lower. In a hostile, disorganized and untidy work environment the turn-over rate of workers was higher than in a normal quiet and orderly environment. Care workers were also less familiar with their clients/patients and quality of care was poor. A large contingent of per diem workers to avoid paying their insurance and other benefits was never a good omen.

STAFF/PATIENT RATIO: Where the ratio of staff to patients was high the quality of care was lower. When one care worker was responsible for a large number of clients, 1/12 (one worker for twelve or more clients). It was then physically impossible to render quality care; Quality care was then degenerated to custodial supervision

COMMUNICATION IN ENGLISH: Where the level of communication in English was poor the quality of care was proportionately lower. Simply put: When a female client /patient calls for the bed—pan and received the urinal, this is not a laughing matter when the need was urgent; it reflected negatively on the quality of care. Social involvement and interactions in reading and games requiring verbal cues are compromised and reflected poorly on the care offered

WAGE SCALE FOR JOB CLASS: Where the wage scale was at or just above the minimum, the quality of care was lower. Incentives often produce positive results as any ranking CEO will readily admit, pun not intended. Higher pay scale seem to reduce absenteeism; work ethics and job satisfaction increase; better trained applicants are attracted and level of care considerably increased. The experience in recruitment of Police Officers is a case in point and mentioned elsewhere in this text.

ODOROUS ENVIRONMENT: Quality of care was low when patients are seen with bed sores, the smell of urine and feces from toilet areas purveyed the atmosphere. This environment was consistent with a poorly administered, poorly supervised, poorly trained staff, and a pay scale at minimum level or just above. In one notable case, the worker saw no harm in inverting the urine collecting bag to drip residual uterine on to the floor daily, insisting that the bag was emptied, emptied but never washed; patient's pillows placed on soiled floor.

DRESS, APPEARANCE AND ENGAGEMENT: The absence of a proper dress code for staff members may be indicative of other omissions and gives a negative impression. Frequent engagements in programs between staff and patients was an indication of a higher level care; these interactions required communicative skills and acceptable level of fluency in English. Clean and orderly attire of clients/patients leave a positive impression on those considering a skilled nursing facility for family members.

AMBIENCE AND *ENVIRONMENT:* A well-attended entrance hall, dining areas, clients' rooms, common areas, and landscaping were all consistent with of a higher level of care. Administrators who paid reasonable attention the physical environment were also attentive to the needs and concerns of the residents. A dimly lighted clients/patients environment enhances a depressive state and viewed negatively.

PLEASANT AND CHEERFUL *STAFF:* When one was able to walk in and out of the facility with impunity, never being challenged by anyone, this experience may portend disaster. However, at the other end of the spectrum in one facility I visited, I was challenged by two guards during the day; there was no receptionist. Before I was able to ask questions, one said to me, "You're in the wrong place. This place ain't for you." I agreed that I was in the wrong place and left without further inquiries. This encounter would merit the lowest score for this entity.

QUALITY CARE ASSESSMENT

Entities/Criteria Rated	Numerical score 1 to 10									
	1	2	3	4	5	6	7	8	9	10
18 to 60 years years: (Lower age, Lower score)										
Eye contact during interview: None to full										
Duration of continuous employment, 1 to 10 years										
Staff/client ratio Available medical coverage and a Rehabilitation consultant										
Ability to communicate in English										
Wage scale for job class										
Odors: Common areas, patient's room, toilet/bath.										
Bed-sores on patients										
Staff/client interaction										
Ambiance (common areas, clients' room, landscape)										
Pleasant and cheerful staff:										

ESTWICK: QUALITY CARE ASSESSMENT TABLE

The highest rating is scored at 100 per cent. You indicate your score for each criteria listed.

TYPICAL JOB DESCRIPTION OF THE HEALTH CARE WORKER

- Shower or bed bath as needed
- Dressing assistance as needed
- Grooming, including skin care, hair care, shampoo, check for skin breakdown
- Foot care/nail care (excludes cutting)
- Oral care, to include brushing and denture care when needed
- Toileting, assisting with bedpan, commode, colostomy, urinal, catheter care as needed with instructions and supervision of nurse in charge
- Transfer assist and bed mobility assist with or without the Hoyer lift
- Ambulation assist, with or without the wheelchair or other assistive devices
- Light meal preparation (in the home)
- Assist in feeding
- Shopping, groceries procurement (in home care)
- Laundering, client's clothing (in home care)
- Light housekeeping around client's quarters (in home care)
- Social or recreational engagement (conversation, games as appropriate)
- Positioning in bed and chair subject to instructions from physical therapist or nurse
- Application of braces and splints, subject to the instructions of physical therapist

OPTIONS IN HEALTH CARE:, In spite of the shortfalls, we are still fortunate to live in a country where there are yet options in respect to choices of health care. It is, however, disturbing that the quality of care is bordering upon the wealth of the individual; this reality taken to its extreme, means that those in the lower-income bracket receive mediocre care and admitted to lower standard institutions. This trend in the delivery of health care is perhaps not unexpected as millions of Americans today are without any health care. The acquisition of long-term care becomes a luxury for most working Americans. Voices of alarm are now being raised as questions of inequity and fairness have reached the doors of Middle America.

Health Care Options for the Purposes of this Book:

- Independent care
- Assisted care
- Skilled nursing care

As discussed earlier, one of the criteria by which a facility is judged is the ratio of caregiver to clients. A ratio of one to five is considered ideal and would allow time for some social interaction with clients. I have seen a ratio as high as one to twelve, which reduces SNC to custodial care. This unacceptable ratio burdens the weakest link in the chain of health care delivery. The rate of absenteeism is disproportionately high and results in poor care of clients. I have given only an overview of the options indicated above. Each facility will establish its unique criteria, but as a "rule of thumb," the following are consistent for admission to most senior care and skilled facilities:

- For independent living: The applicant is expected to be independent in all daily living skills (ADL or activities of daily living). These include bed mobility and transfer activities; independent in toileting, grooming, and self-care; and mentally competent to exercise these activities.
- For assisted living: The critera for this option is variable. In general, the applicant must be independent in most major daily living activities, perhaps requiring assistance in bathing, dressing, grooming, and administration of medication. For example, a post-stroke patient whose only impairment is the functioning of one upper extremity but otherwise capable of independent living. The level of assistance will depend on that which could be safely provided by that institution.

SKILLED NURSING CARE: The applicant must be dependent in several ADL skills, requiring the care and supervision of skilled nursing personnel. Some of the required care may include dehydration, wound care, ventilator, oxygen and respiratory care, special feeding, dialysis, bladder and bowel rehabilitation, mobility and transfer activities. Categories may often be determined by each facility. Some may feel constrained by staffing and the physical structures in place to deal with certain skilled nursing clients and may accept only those clients they feel competent to manage. To be covered as a skilled nursing facility it must be established that the services rendered could only be carried out safely by skilled nursing or skilled rehabilitation personnel. It should be noted that a routine high BP or a stable hemiparesis does not necessarily require skilled nursing for their management.

A question often asked: "What are the objective criteria used to determine acceptance to a skilled nursing facility? *It appears that* more emphasis is placed upon the nursing assessment than on medical status of the clients; this rationale is not without merits since the emphasis in management after admissions is nursing care. The status of patients for whom acute hospital care is not currently indicated, is described as chronic for the most part.

Much reliance is placed on the information obtained from the hospital and community "Patient Review Instrument (A/C-PRI)." One of the categories listed on this review happens to be no. 34, race/ethnic group. There is much controversy about this category because, in the hand of an unscrupulous evaluator, race may be regarded negatively in the selection process of applicants. On the contrary, such information may be useful in treatment and care of the client and serves only his/her best interest.

The experience of one of my patients, regarding admission to a skilled nursing facility leaves many unanswered questions. This patient was denied admission purportedly that the facility was unable to care for her medical needs following a stroke. The residual problems were seizure disorder controlled by medication, the possibility of aspiration because of past history of swallowing difficulties, although the patient fed self without supervision; also that patient was fed via a gastric tube but took supplement liquids by mouth. These were the main concerns of this SNF.

When informed of the patient's denial, there was immediate disbelief. It was interesting that during my discussion with the director of sales, who sent the notice of denial, I sensed a measure of hostility and dismissiveness in her tone and expressions; this prompted me to request her permission to record our discussion, a most unusual request for myself but I sensed the denial of my patient. My request was declined, which I respected. I was not surprised to receive an official denial from this administrator. When I reasoned that this was a skilled nursing facility licensed in the state and benefits from some form of public support, I decided to request an on-site review of my patient by a letter to the CEO of the institution.

SKILLED NURSING: To be denied admission on the premise that a skilled nursing facility is unable to care for the needs of the patient with history of seizure disorder, the possibility of aspiration and receiving supplement feeding via a PEG (a gastric feeding tube) was beyond my comprehension; these needs, in my judgment, are precisely what SNFs are licensed to undertake. The untenable situation is created when the SNF refuses to admit; the hospital refuses to keep the patient; management at home is impossible because of the special needs of the patient. What happens to this human being in a society of great opulence? Refusal to admit for the reasons given by the facility was a justification to question the motives. Also, when race/ethnicity enters into the selection process, questions about fairness are always appropriate.

Why was this patient denied admission? She was treated in an acute care hospital and was discharged to a rehabilitation facility; after she achieved maximum benefit, she was ready for placement. The acute care hospital had judged her condition as chronic, thus no longer required acute hospital care. However, her condition was such that she required skilled nursing intervention that could not be adequately provided in the home environment, but the SNF had just denied her admission, thus the dilemma. It was a situation where a skilled nursing facility was unable or unwilling to do skilled nursing which could not be provided in the home environment and the patient was not suitable for acute hospital care. This patient was fortunate to have an advocate with decades of experience as a rehabilitation specialist/consultant with some knowledge of skilled nursing administration.

The following are excerpts of the letter sent to the executive director/EO of the skilled nursing facility:

I bring this important matter to your attention and respectfully request a review of the denial for admission to your facility. This facility was chosen because of the reputation it has established and its proximity for visitation by close family and friends and the availability of independent living accommodations. I believe the decision to reject this applicant was based on insufficient background information of her current medical status or inadequate interpretation of the information received. I have offered the following in order to supplement the info on which the rejection was based.

Applicant suffered a CVA with left hemiparesis about March 2012; this was followed by episodes of seizure disorder, not uncommon after CVA and quite compatible with SNC; she also had dysphagia, which necessitated a gastric feeding tube; this is also quite a safe device and manageable it all the SNF she has been treated. I am pleased to report that her seizures had been stabilized with medication; she is no longer dysphagic and able to feed herself unsupervised; she also takes liquids by mouth.

There had been no history of aspiration. For your information, the gastric tube remains in place because of the complexity to reinsert in the event of need; this has not occurred since her discharge from hospital. Perhaps her significant problem is that she requires assist for transfers, toilet, and bath; her memory is poor.

In further support of this application, she has received SNC at other facilities and posed no problem which would overwhelm any state-licensed SNF. I submit that to reject anyone for the reasons given may mean to reject most applicants to our SNF.

The admission of anyone implies some risk. I have no doubt that an onsite visit will leave you with an entirely different impression. Regrettably, I sensed this denial during my initial interview with your staff member. This prompted me to ask whether she would wish to be recorded; she declined, and this was respected. I believe to have denied this patient an admission to your facility for reasons stated may be a great miscarriage.

It is my hope that an objective evaluation, taking into account this supportive medical clarification, will be helpful in your decision in this care.

I received a reply from the CEO of the facility shortly after my request for a review. She was gracious, cordial, reasonable and conceded that the information I presented differed from that which was given in the PRI. My patient was reevaluated by the director of nursing and a social workers from the SNF, and they believed the patient was acceptable for their skilled nursing facility, provided financial arrangements were satisfactory. However, she was rejected by the CEO. The absence of an advocate for the interest of your loved ones and the subjectivity in decision making which affect these admissions, are reasons for concern.

Seniors complain about changes in their life style and invasion of their privacy, having to share rooms with others. One senior who had amassed well over $175,000 in savings and contributed generously to the Metropolitan Opera Company, was perturbed that she was now unable to reward a care worker who had consistently and graciously attended to her needs. She said to me, "It's not a nice position to find yourself in." Others seemed to have accepted their station in life in a rather fatalistic manner, believing that fate will determine the future.

Facilities which provide care for seniors vary widely in the services they provide and the amenities they offer. At the lower end of this spectrum, three residents were accommodated in one large dimly lit room with curtain drawn between beds to facilitate some measure of privacy. I was told that these accommodations were for short-term occupants admitted for subacute rehabilitation up to one hundred days, depending on the level of progress. These patients are usually covered by Medicare. Those showing consistent functional improvement may continue their therapy until the level of improvement plateaus. Standard accommodations consisted of two residents to one room. It was interesting to note that most of the residents in these facilities were recipients of Medicaid, the safety net often spoken about. They were converted to this status after exhausting their lifelong savings and other pecuniary possessions. The furnishings in these rooms were functional. The chairs were sturdy and one to each bed; they were not the type one would wish to take home on a dark night to enhance the ambience of his/her abode. There were one chest and one night table for each bed. I do not recall seeing a mirror in these rooms. The presumptive thinking I assumed, seniors had more important problems for their preoccupation than the furnishings in their rooms and certainly not a mirror to see sad faces. The cost for this level of care, including meals, recreational activities, and support services, may range from $275 to $350 each day for SNC. The more upscale facilities charge $540 or higher.

Many residents, with whom I have spoken seem to have acquiesced to this level of care since their basic needs are met, but all things were not all bright and beautiful at some residential facilities. At one facility, although entrance halls seemed immaculate, floors scrupulously clean, shelves in the area were adorned with artifacts from different parts of the country, chairs in the lobby were clean and comfortable, I was very suspicious after being told that I needed an appointment to go beyond that area. However, with my good peripheral vision, keen sense of smell, coupled with my detective instinct, my appointment had already taken place.

As I entered further into the living areas, the sense of an institution, a nursing home, became very apparent. About eight or ten residents were sitting in wheelchairs in a large dayroom, television was on full blast, and one aide worker sat fully asleep along with several residents. There was no doubt that the residents were safe. This was adequate care under the circumstances, custodial care at best. This worker later told me that her relief did not show up, and she was "helping out doing a double." Further into the living/sleeping areas, the smell of urine purveyed the atmosphere through the door of one of the resident's room. It was in fact coming from the toilet/bathroom. I was puzzled that the smell of urine was coming from the bathroom when the patient who occupied the room was not ambulatory and never used the toilet or bath. She was cared for in her bed. Why then was urine spilled over the floor and apparently continued for some time to generate such a strong odor? What transpired was shocking; the patient's urine was collected via an indwelling catheter and a collecting bag as the reservoir. The aide who cared for this patient dutifully emptied the collecting bag with urine into the toilet bowl then inverted the empty collecting bag so that the small amount of residual urine in the catheter/bag drained on the floor daily. Since this toilet/bath was never used by the patient, it was, therefore, never thoroughly cleaned.

The frequency of "double time" is also called into question. What was disconcerting was the fact that this employee was able to perpetuate this unacceptable routine every day without being challenged by a supervisor. The absence of supervision, when many of the care workers were from environments where health codes were less exacting or seldom enforced, was inexcusable. My observation seemed to have negatively characterized the quality of care given to many residents at the lower end of the spectrum.

As I left that institution, I was approached by a gentleman who was also leaving. He was from the city and looking for a home to place his elderly father. He said, "I am very impressed with what I saw."

It was certainly not my role to make recommendations for or against. I asked him whether he had inspected the facility or merely spoken to someone at the entrance desk. I suggested that he should inspect the dayroom, dining rooms, patient's room, toilet/bath and talk to a few employees and find out the staff-client ratio. He may then be able to make an independent decision. Talking to an administrator was the least reliable or objective way to assess the quality care in any given institution. This encounter prompted me to establish a comprehensive quality care assessment table to evolve a mechanism for judging quality care at a given institution. One must live in a house to know where it leaks.

I also visited facilities at the upper end of the spectrum which may best be described as lavish. The ambience was reminiscent of a five-star hotel. The familiar nursing-home odor was absent, bath/toilet were no exception. The ratio of staff to clients was said to be one is to seven, one aide worker to seven residents. Except for those patients covered by Medicare and receiving physical therapy, private patients paid about $465-$540 per day for skilled nursing care to remain in these institutions. Some do not accept Medicaid recipients, which probably excludes the "47 percent." Such expenditure for health care alone is an outrage to most middle-income Americans. Care in some of these facilities was no better than care at home when this could be adequately provided and at a lower cost. For many patients with dementia, the care was virtually custodial. For those whose problems were marginal, there was inadequate individual stimulation since most of the activities were conceptualized for a large group, with or without dementia. The cost to enter some independent care facility in New York State is startling and prohibitive for most citizens. To these charges, there are additional state occupancy charge of 6.8 percent, an additional charge of $34,000 entrance charge for the second occupant, monthly fee of $870. The irony, these occupancy charges are assessed for skilled nursing care patients who are in need of institutional care and supervision. They are not residents of resort hotels; they are sick and disabled who are in need of care, professional nursing care; yet they are taxed for the care they receive. Where are the merciful?

Accommodations		Entry Fees	Monthly Fees
1 BR	Balcony	$474,000	$3,600
1 BR	Balcony	$457,040	$3,600
1 BR	Balcony	$473,000	$3,680
2 BR	(1,030 sq. ft.)	$638,280	$4,090
BR	(1,147 sq. ft.)	$761,810	$4,420
2 BR	(1,190 sq. ft.)	$770,610	$4,420
2 BR	(1,586 sq. ft.)	$1,025,890	$5,155
3 BR	(1,900 sq. ft.)	$1,224,245	$5,637

The cost varies from facility to facility and from state to state and, in some instances, relates to the services they provide. Facility at one state could be entered for as little as $175,000 with a monthly rental fee of $2,000 with no state occupancy charges (tax).

AFFORDABLE SENIOR CARE: Affordable senior care has become a utopia for the many citizens who desperately needs it, and the prime reason for this shift is the extraordinary cost. By my calculation, a senior citizen may be expected to spend well over $100,000 per year for accommodation in the average skilled nursing facility (SNF). Institutions are known to charge a single senior patient as much as $187,000 per year plus 6.8 percent as "cash receipt assessment" extracted by some state departments of health in order to receive SNC; to characterize such payments as unconscionable may be an understatement when one considers that over 80 percent of working Americans never earn this salary per year. To add a dubious exclusiveness, some institutions refuse Medicaid patients, yet all of these institutions directly or indirectly receive some form of state or federal assistance. Why should anyone desperately in need of continuing medical/nursing care be required to pay what amounts to be a state tax assessment which I am told may be refundable?

I was troubled to learn that the commissioner of health for one state had authorized a fee of 6.8 percent for the SNC of patients/clients who had suffered a major medical event. The victim continued to require skilled nursing care for residual deficits which could not be given at his home. His medical problems were too complex to be managed at home, and they were not at the level for continued hospital care. They fell within the province of SNC. A room in the best hotel could not provide for such demanding medical/nursing attention.

My discussions with a director of nursing at one institution had confirmed that their patients/clients were in fact receiving SNF: "All eighty-four beds are skilled nursing, they are not custodial."

With this assurance and with the medical/nursing needs of these patients, why then should they be taxed for accommodation under these circumstances? It is very tempting to assume that the state as also complicit in this unwarranted escalation of cost in the delivery of health care to its senior citizens who seem to have no advocate in this regard.

One senior citizen who was admitted to an institution designated as a skilled nursing facility (SNF) was surprised that 6.8 percent was added to his $15,000 monthly charges for care. The patient suffered a stroke and required near maximum assistance for his care. He had frequent seizures and required monitoring and stabilization of his seizure medications. He had difficulty swallowing and had to be fed through a tube inserted into the abdomen. He had developed an ulcer over the heel and this required professional care. The blood pressure which was unstable had to be monitored. Clearly, these are conditions which require SNC; they are not conditions to be treated in a room at a resort hotel or at home. For this patient, a billing plan was contrived so that instead of being billed for skilled nursing (SN), he was billed merely for his room rent as though he occupied living quarters in a residential hotel. Nothing was mentioned about skilled nursing.

The institution had nothing to do with these tax assignments; they merely carry out the mandate of the respective state. This type of billing I believe, was contrived to allow the state to collect 6.8 percent on his monthly payments, which quickly exhausted his limited assets. In order to justify such tax/fee for SNC, I conjecture that the skilled nursing facility had reduced itself to the status of a rooming house for the purpose of billing which then billed for what amounts to room rent. It is troubling that a state would subscribe to such a scheme. Such tax as I see it, on one who is already burdened by illness, seemed hard to justify. The scheme adapted to bill for a room instead of billing for SNC justified the added cost of 6.8 percent extracted by the state Department of Health. How does one justify billing for one room, $15,000 a month and then the billing for a two bedroom apartment in the same institution at $5,000 a month? Answers to these questions remain inexplicable at best. Clearly, another case of a "mathematical absurdity."

CHARGES AT SOME FACILITIES: The following represent charges covering thirty-eight days at one skilled care facility:

Room charges (7 days)	$3,461.57
State assessment (tax 6.8%)	$235.41
Room charges (31 days)	$15,329.81
State assessment (tax 6.8%)	$1,042.53
Total charges (thirty-eight days)	$20,069,323

At this rate, a client would need $16,372.34 each month and $196,468.08 each year. What percent of the American population could afford such cost for one person who probably earned one quarter of that amount annually during the working years? I know of several families who were unable to save that amount during their entire working years. A reasonable person may describe such cost as outrageous which only millionaires can afford. Such obscene rates for health care far exceed the annual income of virtually all mid-income Americans, many of whom were unable to initiate or maintain a long-term insurance policy and are ineligible for Medicaid coverage. One official was quick to explain that "once one is admitted, no one is thrown out." The question then becomes "Who do they admit, and what are the contracts for admission?"

Contract for admission to many elder care facilities varies and not always an easy matter. Many seniors chose the entire elder care package where they receive varying levels of care during their lifetime. The usual procedure, they are first admitted to the independent care unit where residents are able to function independently, except for contracted meals and housekeeping arrangements. When they decline and unable to carry out their daily functions, they may then qualify for residence in the assisted care unit or the skilled care unit, according to the level of their functional needs. There are, however, occasions for direct admission to any one unit. The admission policy of many facilities call for preapproval of financial status before one is considered a candidate.

You must submit the following:

- Evidence about your equity in your principal residence
- CDs and savings
- Stocks and other investments savings bonds
- Evidence of your social security benefits
- retirement and pension benefits
- Life insurance
- Long-term insurance

Statement about your assets must be substantiated by letters from your tax preparer or attorney. I am told that if your financial data are not approved, "your application is dead." The next hurdle to overcome is the entrance fee; this is the initial payment in order to access a bungalow, an apartment, or a studio, according to your ability to pay and the availability of these accommodations. This down payment ranges from $475,000 to over $1 million plus a monthly rental fee from $3,600 to $5,000 at some institution. Keep in mind you are paid no interest on this down payment and are required to pay an additional monthly rental occupancy tax of 6.8 percent as assessed by the state Department of Health. Your down payment is said to be kept in escrow and returned to you when you leave or to your estate when you expire. The institution keeps all the accrued interests and dividends. It is a virtually interest-free loan to the institution. It is, therefore, very simplistic to assert that "no one is thrown out if unable to pay after your admission."

Some institutions have policies which will allow them to defer payments in the event resident is unable to make monthly payments. They will in fact deduct payments from any entrance fee held in escrow. With such large entrance payments, institutions certainly will have several years of financial coverage held in escrow from which to draw in the event of inability to meet monthly payments. The claim of allowing residents who are unable to pay to remain has to be taken with some trepidation. It is estimated that the $1 million on entrance, held in escrow for 5 years and invested at 5 percent interest rate, will earn the institution $250,000 in addition to the huge sums already paid by residents for monthly rentals. One financial manager at a large investment company sees this as "an ingenious scheme because if a resident choses to leave after five years or expires, the institution reaps an additional $250,000 or more, with prudent investments in today's market." Most institutions are quite open in their policies and disclosures but promises "not to throw you out" have to be carefully read and understood. Applicants must read and fully understand the contracts they sign; this may require interpretation by an attorney.

I have spoken to relatives who found it necessary to hire additional caregiver for their loved ones so that they receive acceptable care, although they pay $500.00 a day for skilled nursing care. The charges for SNC continue to rise in the name of inflation which did not occur nor were wages for workers increased during that period.

Some seniors expressed the view that some staff in physical rehabilitation tended to be very aggressive and demanding; I do concur that some were better suited for younger clients in a sports-related gymnasium. They seem to forget that seniors are slower to heal, require a special approach physically and psychologically. The increments of improvement in the senior clients are often very miniscule. Seniors require more encouragement to continue the course of therapy. They have to be reassured that they are in fact improving. The latter concept is familiar. A beautiful young married female, although aware of her beauty, feels neglected and disavowed if her spouse never reassures her. With most seniors, the intensity of therapy has to be gradual and with some rest periods. These can be achieved and yet fulfill the minimum time requirements for Medicare coverage. Many seniors are written off and characterized as having achieved maximum benefit. More often, it is the therapist showing his/her impatience for the slow rate in progress of the senior, who is also burdened by many comorbid issues unknown to the zealous and aggressive therapist. A common error is to set goals which had never been achieved by patients prior to admission. A good history on admission would have disclosed this so that realistic goals are set.

I have often intervened when the course of therapy had been abruptly halted because of inappropriate goals set by a therapist. Independent ambulation is hardly an appropriate short-term goal for a hemiplegia, unable to sit or stand because of trunk weakness and weakness in the lower extremities. A more realistic short-term goal should be trunk strengthening, sitting balance and tolerance, standing and weight shifting, ambulation in the parallel bars. Ultimately, the long-term goal may be gait training and independent ambulation or ambulation with assistive device. This misstep in priority has been one reason for shortchanging of seniors in the course of their rehabilitation management. They are precipitously discharged when they still have rehabilitation potentials, keeping in mind that patients achieve their full potentials in their home and natural environment. Physical rehabilitation of seniors requires personnel with special temperament, those with empathy, patience, and slow to anger; those who can distinguish plateauing from a slow and sustained rate of improvement as observed in many seniors.

I have received reports from therapy staff that: "They (seniors) complain about everything, it doesn't matter what I do." My usual retort has sided with seniors because I believe that for many seniors, this is a way to vents their frustrations, having been confined for extended periods and having no one with whom to express their emotions. Therapy staff, who have the freedom to go and come and make their own decisions, must learn to deal with this "annoyance." It was my judgment that the ambience of the institution did not always translate to quality rehabilitation. This was always the domain of the individual therapist. Other problems commonly experienced by seniors during the course of their rehabilitation are constipation and ascending urinary tract infection. Inadequate fluid intake (water), inadequate roughage in diet, lack of physical exercise, many seniors ignore their urge to use the toilet, these are well known contributing factors to constipation. For many seniors, use of the bedpan is another inhibiting factor often overlooked. It is not enough to ask the client whether there was a BM; the care worker/aide must verify. Seniors on aspirin regime have experienced GI bleeding which was not diagnosed for weeks because the care worker failed to note the change in color of client's stool. One senior was found to be lethargic during her physical therapy program; she was in fact severely anemic. Her physical therapist had failed to connect her lethargy with her underlying medical problem, anemia. The therapist only saw one side of the coin. Urinary tract infection is another medical problem often overlooked by nursing staff who should be the "gatekeeper." The inexperienced physical therapist and occupational therapist should hardly be expected to recognize these often subtle medical problems experienced by seniors under their care. Urinary tract infection, if ignored, may result in an acute medical emergency leading to the demise of the patient.

One patient whom I have followed had complained of "pain in her butt" for several weeks. When I examined the patient, her problem was quite obvious; it was a perianal infection and was ignored because the care worker who examined the client reported that she saw nothing unusual, yet the client continued to complain. This problem was due to poor or lack of adequate perianal care in a patient who was totally dependent for this service; nursing supervision was also inadequate. This patient continued to attend therapy with this infection and complained of feeling cold. She ultimately became very lethargic and diaphoretic (sweating). It was only then that the patient was examined by a nurse and transferred for acute medical care with the nebulous diagnosis of altered mental status, meaning "I don't know what the problem is." I view "altered mental status" as a clinical sign which reflects an underlying problem; admittedly, the problem may often be very obscured. The use of a wet towel from running water at the sink without use of soap or a wash basin is inadequate toilet care for the senior, and this is routine at some SCF. Some cleansing cloth in use are only time savers and give a false sense of proper toileting.

A definitive diagnosis for my patients was made on admission after a simple urinalysis and blood review. Here again, there was a total disconnect by the nursing staff and the rehabilitation staff. The total patient was ignored and seen only as a rehabilitation subject. Regrettably, I have found these "disconnect" pervasive at several institutions. Daily living activities seem to terminate at the door of the rehabilitation department. The ward staff and care workers are unwilling or unable to carry over that which was accomplished in the rehabilitation department. A common infraction is the lack of proper positioning in bed to which I have referred earlier in this book.

A similar disconnect was observed in toilet training. Patients who were encouraged to sit on the commode after each heavy meal three times daily have been able to regulate their movements and avoiding the unpleasant and embarrassing experience of soiling themselves and diapers. They often express disdain when this is allowed to happen.

Whenever I participate in in-service training, I have often emphasized: "That staff at all institutions are employed only because there are clients/patients to be served and without whom, there would be no need for their employment." With this preamble, I expect the highest respect, empathy, and consideration given to all clients/patients, irrespective of their mental, physical, or social status.

It should never be assumed that all physically disabled clients are devoid of social, physical, and intellectual capacity, therefore would not perceive or recognize those actions which are demeaning and dehumanizing. I have seen the regular use of the commode abandoned by caregivers with the full sanction of supervisors because to use this would be inconvenient for the care worker; this is done with a disregard for the respect of clients who preferred the use of this appliance. It is regrettable that those clients whose cognition may be intact but motor functions compromised may fall victim of these wanton abuse which I have exposed here. It is hoped that institutions will find more acceptable ways to address what has become an institutional culture and causes indelible harm to clients/patients. I make reference here to the entire regimen of toileting and "toilet training." This neglect on the part of caregivers is compounded by the inordinately long waiting period before their diapers are changed.

I have observed that in spite of clearly written prescription for commode activities after meals, care workers consistently allowed clients to soil themselves because they claim "this is easier to deal with" than placing clients on the commode. These patients never benefit from the commode training they received in Occupational Therapy. One patient who requested the commode at 12:30 p.m. after her meal was told "someone was coming over." When the care worker arrived at 1:30 p.m., the embarrassed patient had already soiled herself. The sphincter of the elderly is unable to resist the challenge of nature for such extended period. I emphasized that many of these seniors, who are branded as incontinent, do have normal elimination functions. They simply cannot get to their destination, the toilet, in a timely manner. Whenever I deal with this issue, I would pointedly ask the caregiver,

"How many hours could you tolerate fecal contamination lying in your bed?" I believe when this is made personal, the question is clearer.

After eight weeks as a resident at one of the best care facilities in the state and at considerable cost, I was alarmed and disappointed to note that my patient had developed a decubitus over the lateral (outer) surface of the right heel; this extremity was not affected by a recent stroke. This development was noteworthy because the occurrence of her CVA had been about eight months prior; throughout this period, she had been in hospital, home care, and other health-related facility. Any reasonable person may ask, "Why has she developed decubitus in one of the best-run facilities in the state, which was expressly selected to avoid these occurrences?" My answer to the question was stated previously.

Ulcers and skin breakdown are not uncommon in patients who are sedentary, bed and wheelchair-bound, not receiving any structured physical therapy care, and are neglected. I believe these patients should automatically be placed on a "high risk status" for decubitus ulcer.

My recommendation to the staff: "The best way to treat the decubitus ulcer in the adult care community is to prevent it from occurring." The prevalence of decubitus in any institution is often an indication of poor quality care and supervision, tantamount to neglect. A high rate in occurrence of decubitus ulcers is directly related to poor level of care. There is an interesting paradox: "The higher the cost the poorer the care." Paying over $500 a day, there should be no ulcers and reasons given for their occurrences are not tenable but simply justify these infractions.

Simply put, "Ischemic/pressure ulcers are the direct result of local pressure and/or friction to an existing vulnerable skin and subcutaneous area and often associated with neglect. Other contributing factors may include poor nutritional state, the presence of local edema which increases cell/ capillary distance; circulation deficiency from any cause reduces oxygen, electrolytes, and vital nutriments to issue. Friction is believed to cause shearing effect on peripheral vessels with stretching and compromise the local circulation." Kosiak believes most pressure ulcers are preventable (*Archives of Physical Medicine and Rehabilitation* 42:19-29 1961).

Patients' fees allocated for maintenance of areas of glitter and glamor may be better used in decubitus prevention, including the use of special mattresses and a lower worker-clients ratio. Administrators should be reminded that these institutions exist primarily for the clients/patients they have the privilege to serve. No institution will exist in the absence of these citizens. The 80/20 rule of the Affordable Care Act should be applied to these institutions. Whenever fees are raised by institutions, this increment does not necessarily reflect a parallel increase in the quality of patients' care nor an increase in wages for the caregivers. It may, however, reflect the end-of-year bonuses for top-level administrators.

PROGRAM FOR STAFF CONVENIENCE: "What good is served if man lives only for himself?" I have used this paraphrased quotation after observing staff effecting plans and programs for the convenience of the staff, with only incidental consideration for the patients whom they serve. This observation was notable when I served as a UNDP (Tokten) consultant in one of the Caribbean/South America countries after a patient arrived at the emergency room about 3:00 p.m. that day. *I was called to treat the patient who* was said to have a laceration. When I arrived at the cubicle, there was no patient but instead a member of the cleaning staff assiduously mopping the floor and dusting. There was no other cubicle available. By this time, my patience was wearing thin. The young man had a protrusion of his patella (kneecap) from a laceration caused by a cut steel drum.

I asked the worker, "Why isn't the patient in the cubicle?"

She calmly said to me, "He got to wait outside till me finish cleaning the floor because me stop work at four o'clock."

I told her, "The patient had a serious problem and had to be seen immediately."

She was unimpressed and said, "I got to finish the floor."

I had her out of the cubicle within seconds and proceeded to attend to the young man who was in pain and bleeding. I had the knee x-rayed to rule our fractures; the wound was cleaned, irrigated, antibiotics applied profusely locally. The patella was replaced, deep non-resolvable sutures were applied, restrictive pressure dressing applied, anti-tetanus and systemic antibiotics administered and prescribed. He was put on a non-weight-bearing program and instructions to return in a week or before if he had increased pain, swelling, discoloration, or fever. On subsequent visits several years later, I tried to make contact with this patient, but he was said to have left the country and living in Canada. I had never replaced a patella before. Fortunately, there were no fractures. It was only a matter of cleaning the wound and closing the laceration. I never had the opportunity to see the long-term outcome of my work. This was probably an orthopedic intervention, but I was the only medical personal there. This cleaning staff exemplifies the extreme in serving the interest of the caregivers, terminating her work at 4:00 p.m. There was no consideration given to the suffering of the patient; no human good was being served by her action. I have seen similar conduct in institutions I visited in the United States when the first meal of the day, breakfast, was served to my patient in his room. Breakfast arrived at 8:00 a.m.; the patients should be served routinely at that time; Instead, the food languished while the caregiver spends hours attending to everything, except assisting the patient with his meals; when served breakfast (cooked cereal, egg, tea) was cold, and the time was approaching 10:30 a.m. In two hours, it will be lunchtime. Cold breakfast is the least appetizing for anyone. Some clients/patients refuse to eat and unwilling or unable to express their dissatisfaction. Nothing in this scenario was conceptualized for the convenience or well-being of the client. "This is how it's done." The routine of immediate serving described, works well in home care and would no doubt work well for select patients in institutions. Patients should be placed on the commode immediately after meals as part of the toilet training routine. After these needs (breakfast then commode) are satisfied, the task of washing and bathing patient may then be initiated. This routine has been effective with paraplegics and has worked in home care because it is conceptualized entirely for the patient and not for the convenience of the staff. However, staff insists that it is easier changing soiled diaper in bed than placing patient on the commode. This is clearly another area of service where the interest of patients is subordinated to the interest and convenience of the staff.

A more acceptable alternative which was very successful in home care is to feed the client/patient as soon as breakfast arrives while it is yet warm; after breakfast, the patient may then be placed on the commode. This is the best way to establish a bowel regimen if done routinely. Following this routine, client/patient may then embark on routine morning wash-up and oral hygiene. The existing system seems flawed and serves more the interest and convenience of the staff. I do concede that in order to function effectively, some consideration must be given to staffing and their needs, but there seems to be an overreach in this direction. A balance must be evolved, but when the administration and the care workers see only justification in their actions, there can be no effective change to an entrenched philosophy, it then becomes "It is my opinion, therefore our belief." Who are the advocates for these clients/patients whose care are entrusted in these institutions and their caregivers?

Health care in the home environment under certain conditions may provide a more desirable outcome for some seniors than that provided in many skilled care facilities, notwithstanding the glitter they may provide at their entrance halls. One resident, struggling to find words for her preference for home care, after spending a month in a skilled care facility, said, "Home is where I belong. it is my home." These words by one who "lived on both sides of the street" were powerful and meaningful to me. A change of surrounding, especially for a senior citizen, could be challenging and unsettling; the physical orientation is completely changed; the once familiar corner in the house or apartment where she had coffee and watched the birds building their nests was not there; friends and acquaintances no longer exist. The depth of their anguish over changes that seem insignificant to many is difficult or impossible to fathom. A change in the lives of senior citizens from living at home to living within the confines of the best long term care facility is hard to accept. The cost of institutional care is by far *greater than the cost of living at home and the care at home is more individualized. Clients in SNFs who were continent were* allowed to soil themselves because a care worker was unable or unwilling to assist them in a timely manner; she had a patient ratio of one to ten.

I concede that there are some notable advantages to institutional care, and these have to be taken into account when deciding on the ideal environment for your loved ones. It is always best to make the decisions when possible, with the full acquiescence of your loved ones. Institutional residence eliminates the maintenance of a home with all the countless and varied responsibilities—repairs, heat, light, mortgage payments, and the inevitable taxes and insurance. Institutional care may also provide easier access to professional services (medical and nursing personnel) in the event of medical emergencies. It assures the continuity of care because of the larger pool of care workers present at any given time during a twenty-four-hour period. In spite of all these advantages, there are those who continue to show an overwhelming preference for care in their homes. There was something intangible in their reasoned preference and decision.

FOOD SERVICES: I observed food preparation and service at senior care facilities because these often escape the attention of clients, their family, and inspectors. The preoccupation seems to be focused less on food selection and preparation and more on other issues, including cost. I do not minimize the need and importance of food inspections; they may reveal alarming conditions which are injurious to the health and safety of patients/clients and employees of these institutions; inspections should be encouraged, and more nonscheduled inspections should be made. There is, however, great skepticism when inspectors seem more interested in protecting the vices of the institutions rather than the interest of residents. The importance of food selection and preparation deserve more scrutiny than is presently given. It is one thing to have a good food manager, but it is more important to have a good chef. Many routine inspections fail to observe the quality of the produce being prepared and the way they are prepared.

The experience of one patient who suffered a stroke was quite telling; in addition to the left extremity weakness, he had minimal to moderate difficulty in swallowing. In order to facilitate his nutritional intake, a feeding device was improvised so that liquids and medications may be given as needed. He had progressed from pureed to minced food by mouth. However, when minced or chopped meat was served, he refused to eat. The exception to his refusal was when fish was served. This aroused my suspicion that perhaps there may be other factors responsible for the inability or refusal to eat consistently. My suspicion was confirmed after it was observed that the patient was able to chew, swallow, and digest meat when this was selected and prepared at home.

The speech therapist who also evaluates problems relating to chewing and swallowing was consulted. I received more opinions than I expected: "The patient had a swallowing problem," which was well known. "His appetite is poor, he is probably depressed. It may be his denture." (He had none).

The consultant was willing to place the blame entirely on the patient who had little to say in all these deliberations. The fact being, this patient was transferred to the institution at considerable cost each day with the high hopes of finding an institution that would serve his needs. There was the implicit assumption that those responsible for selection and preparation of meals were infallible. Hence, the focus was exclusively on clients/patient.

I took a different view and decided to test the quality of the food being served to this patient; the texture of the meat served was a fiasco. I commented about the quality of the meat served and the food in general. The following week, turkey drumstick, along with vegetables, was prepared by the family at home for the patient. The result was remarkable. The patient drank the broth, chewed the meat, and had little or no residue in his mouth after his meal. My impression was confirmed, that the selection and preparation of food at the institution left much to be desired. Some meals seem to have been served directly from the butchers, others cooked the previous year. Among the worst prepared meals there must be one which was at least satisfactory. My exhortation would be: "Reach out and express your pleasure and satisfactions; it may inspire positive change in future meals.

SENIOR CARE PHYSICIANS: In former years, any licensed physician was recruited to serve in senior care facilities (SNF and assisted care). In recent years, the trend has shifted so that these physicians are expected to have formal training or experience in geriatric care or certification in geriatric medicine. My friend who was the director of a skilled nursing facility offered me a position at the facility. I declined his offer, telling him that I did not have the training or experience to fill the position as a geriatric physician. He assured me that my internal medicine and physical rehabilitation background were adequate if supplemented by some in service courses. "The job is easy," he said. "You don't have to kill yourself to do a good job."

My experience, however, showed a different picture. In many respects, the work was very challenging, demanding, and required intuitive skill and time to penetrate the minds of senior citizens, many of whom were unable or unwilling to give information necessary to arrive at a working diagnosis. To make a diagnosis, the physician must rely on the history from the patient with the findings on physical examination. Fortunately, most seniors entering the SNF come with a working diagnosis.

Titration of medication: The effective dose and time of administration of some medication could be very challenging, especially medications with sedating effects. I have seen a post-stroke patient with history of seizure disorder on whom the physician was unable to arrive at a dose/time schedule which kept patient awake during the day. In spite of this difficulty, a neurological consultation was never sought. My thought was that this task was clearly beyond the scope of the geriatrician. It was perhaps easier and safer to keep the patient like a zombie, sedated for most of the day, than to risk the onset of a seizure episode. This thinking and action made life for the physician easier, no disturbing calls for unexpected seizure activities during the days or nights. This approach supports my friend's view of an easy job. This, however, resulted in an untenable situation for the patient who was unable to have food by mouth, and a feeding device had to be put in place to maintain the nutritional needs of the patient. What was especially troubling, the patient was unable to participate in his physical rehabilitation programs, the prime reason for his admission to the subacute program. Managing this patient, even in SNF, was not an easy task. I believe most geriatric physicians ventured into the specialty because of their interest in caring for the medical needs of seniors. They did not elect this specialty as an easy one, affording them time to take the children to after-school soccer games and the like. They saw it as a vocation, not as a career.

"Words of Wisdom to New Doctors," (Professor Emeritus Henry Fraser of the University of the West Indies) emphasizing the difference between one's vocation and job, addressing the 2013 graduates, "I say vocation and not a career because if you see it as a vocation, a calling by God to his services, you will be richly rewarded in all the ways that really matter, not just a comfortable living. If you see it just as a career, to earn a fat salary and a BMW, you will never know the joys that true medical service brings."

PUBLIC REPORTS: The operations at one large health care conglomerate were recently exposed to public view; what was seen and heard were shocking to many viewers. However, I had become immune by similar conduct at other health care facilities; for me, it was simply a rerun. The care given to seniors is as good as the people and institutions which provide them. I have expressed empathy with caregivers throughout this publication; they bear the brunt in the delivery of health care to seniors and others. I regard them as the front line of defense. When this line becomes vulnerable without secondary support, the system will collapse and the patients will suffer. Having expressed my support for caregivers of the system, I also see opportunities for improving the delivery of care without increasing the traditional workload of caregivers.

In some institutions, there appear to be absence of structure and consistency in programs they offer. Programs well described and articulated were seldom carried out and seemed fictional. It was a classic description of what should be done but was never carried out as described. Lofty goals were set for individual patient and groups which, in my view, were not achievable. Goals should be reasonably achievable, and when achieved, new goals are set. For my stroke patients, short-term goal may be to improve strength, range, bed mobility, and sitting balance. After these are achieved, I may progress to intermediate goals and long-term goals. A patient whose weakness is so profound that he is unable to use his extremity or turn in his bed, setting an immediate goal for ambulation is unrealistic. Many of the problems observed, however, were more fundamental than the setting of goals; they are related to job description for employees so that each worker knows the reason for his/her employment. On more than one occasion, I heard employees bitterly protesting to supervisors, "This is not my job!" apparently not knowing all the tasks she was employed to carry out during the course of the day. She had completed her morning tasks and felt that that was all she was expected to do for the morning. As it transpired, the hiring process was so constricted and vague that the new worker was never properly orientated about her job description. Some institutions have shared the job description with the workers to avoid such confusion.

Staff Interaction With Clients: Ideally, there should always be opportunities for care staff to interact with clients/patients outside of the routine work assignment. It is not sufficient to leave this important social intervention to the discretion of caregivers; it should be assigned. There are few interventions more stimulating than the presence of staff sitting among clients, talking, laughing, and the like. Although this is a passive exercise so far as workers are concerned, the mere presence of these workers is stimulating and beneficial to both staff and their clients/patients. When this could not be accomplished, the worker/client ratio was disproportionately high; a ratio of one to ten was found to be too high to accomplish this goal. A ratio of one to six or lower was compatible with the fulfillment of this schedule.

The association of care workers with clients—perhaps watching an old movie, listening to familiar music, chatting informally, participating in games—create an environment of care, trust, and camaraderie. Although this may be outside the principal task of caregivers, they are within their job description. They are justified and provide a respite for care workers from their core responsibilities. This alternative is to be preferred than having patients seated in crowded hallways or to have six wheelchairs crowded in a sitting room intended for six or eight occupants without wheelchairs. Unfortunately, absence of appropriate space at some facilities is a structural problem and difficult to remedy without great cost; they reflect poor planning with no thought given to the recreational needs of seniors who are sometimes packed like sardines in these rooms. Our prison population today enjoys larger space for the recreational needs of inmates. I am told that, in some instances, these are mandated by the courts. How about our senior citizens? It is often more feasible to add an entire memory care unit, as an addition to the original structure, than to create a proper recreation room to accommodate seniors entrapped in their domicile.

Productive Work: It is well known that a happy worker is usually a productive worker. Institutions serve the interest of patients because that has been their mission and the reason that they exist. The mission of service can only be accomplished with the cooperation and productivity of its staff. My survey has disclosed that health care workers, although at the bottom of the wage scale, were also concerned about issues outside the umbrella of wages. They had questions about eating and toilet facilities for staff at some institutions; these necessities seem to have received only second thoughts in the planning of some institutions and are now here to haunt them. Without properly structured accommodations, workers are sometimes seen eating a full meal at their desks which some prefer to the accommodation set aside for this purpose; I was told that some workers (RNs, LPNs) prefer eating at their work table to save time because they work a sixteen-hour shift without much time off to eat. Some workers eat at a corner in the patients' dining room. I have seen the odd worker standing and eating; I am sure this was their preference. I take cognizance of these conditions only because they do have influence on productivity and, consequently, care of seniors. I look upon the entire process of eating as one of the pleasures of life; for many, it is also a social intervention. I believe health care workers and all workers should be provided with at least a semblance of this process so that they enjoy the act of eating. Adjustments of structural deficiencies, where feasible, to accommodate the needs of workers would certainly enhance not only the working environment of caregivers but also the quality of care they deliver.

Administrators and Institutions who actively strive to maximize the quality of care they deliver to their charges sometimes at great odds with their executives, should be commended. These administrators do their best to serve the needs of people, their patients; their employment stems from the fact that these patients and institutions exist. The philosophy of chief executives seems to focus more on interest and dividends of shareholders and their own salaries and bonuses.

In some occurrences reported by the press, the interests of patients are incidental and secondary. Ultimately, institutions which serve the needs of patients will prevail in spite of this divergence of interest. There are, however, administrators who spend countless hours formulating plans to improve the care of patients; they meet with advocates, inviting comments and opinions. I have seen administrators visiting local areas of care, not relying entirely on reports of supervisors; they should also be placed in the column as the "foot soldiers" who maintain the "pyramid" described in this publication. The tasks of these administrators are far more difficult because they have to serve and please two masters: the patient population and their advocates on one hand, and their chief executives on the other, the latter often totally ignorant of operation in the battleground, day-to-day patient's care.

For many seniors who express their concern about medical records and the course of their care/treatment, I assure you that most institutions stand ready to share with you or your advocates information relevant to your care and treatment. Institutions now share your medical information with other institutions and with many government agencies. Gone are the days when your medical records were the exclusive domain of institutions. Remember, you have paid for the tests and consultations related to your care directly or through your insurance carriers. Access to your records from physicians or institutions is now perceived to be your right. You should not hesitate to request them if there is a need.

The law is clear in reference to access of your medical information and section 18 of the Public Health Law outlines procedures, whereby patients may apply by written request for access to their records. Requests may also be made to your family physician, and in the case of institutions, this may be made through the director or the keeper of records at the institution. The law also allows a time limit within which you may have the opportunity to view your records. Written copies may be obtained through written application. Physicians and institutions are sometimes reluctant to pass on any information to patients; these denials are not uncommon especially with immigrants, minorities, and those who it is perceived may not be knowledgeable enough to challenge or to raise questions. Minority patients often fall in this category of denials.

There may be charges for service. In the event your application is denied, you have the option of appealing to the state Department of health.

Long-Term Insurance (LTI)

I have highlighted long-term insurance (LTI) because it is playing a very important role in the delivery of care, and senior citizens are becoming more interested in this type of insurance coverage. Long-term coverage may determine the quality and duration of institutional care a senior receives. It may also preclude seniors converting to Medicaid status due to depletion of their lifelong assets.

What is long-term care? These are contracted insurance policies sold widely by a number of insurance carriers in North America and the United Kingdom. These contracts enable the insured to pay for their extended care (long term) after certain health conditions are met. It must be understood that these policies do not cover the primary medical care which may be covered by Medicare or Medicaid insurance. Long-term care insurance generally covers individuals who are unable to perform their activities of daily living (ADL) in total or in part. Some of these activities include dressing, grooming, toileting, getting in and out of bed, transferring, walking, etc. The insured may require assisted or total care; this assistance may be given in the home by an aide or in an institution. Although a relatively small number of seniors are presently insured, it is estimated that about 60 percent of those over sixty-five years may require some form of LTC over their life span; a significant number would be below this age group. About 40 percent of those currently receiving long-term care are between eighteen and sixty-four years. Diseases, such as multiple sclerosis, and other early onset illnesses render the insured more likely to access LTC coverage at earlier age. In the normal course of events, Medicaid, often referred to as the welfare program, may provide long-term care benefits for applicants who are qualified.

In spite of some reservation, these policies may cover a wide range of conditions which may occur during the life of the insured. Coverage may also include Alzheimer's care, respite care, day care, home care, assisted care, hospice care, and others. It may cover for a live-in caregiver, housekeeper, private duty nurse, coverage to the maximum limit of your contract. One should note that these benefits may not be applicable in all policies. It is therefore important that those who negotiate an individual contract should be aware that there may be restrictions applied.

They must also be mindful that those who represent the insurance carriers, the agents, may not disclose many of the roadblocks one may encounter when it is time to access your policy. I therefore urge you to read, especially the fine prints which tend to benefit the insurance carriers and, therefore, not in their interest to illuminate. The fine prints under certain circumstances are intended to obfuscate and deceive; the smaller the prints, the bigger the obfuscation and should prompt the curiosity of the applicant to get out the magnifying glasses. In these circumstances, I also urge applicants to be paranoid; your paranoia may be your only protection against misinformation and deception.

Long-term insurance carriers may discourage some seniors from enrollment. This is done by including in their application forms certain medical conditions peculiar to seniors, which will automatically exclude them or cover them at exorbitant premiums. Younger applicants are preferred. They are less likely to qualify or apply for health care benefits; they are less prone to many of the ailments experienced by seniors. When benefit payments to the insured are low and premium payments rocketing, insurance carriers are assured of higher levels of cash retention and bigger bonuses for top-level administrative staff.

One applicant complained that he was rejected or placed in the highest level premium payment category because he indicated on his application that he had arthritis and spinal stenosis, although he never had any symptoms. The applicant was given this information by his physician, who explained that it was an incidental finding revealed after he had fallen off his bicycle and had an x-ray evaluation of his spine; it required no treatment. This applicant was sixty-eight years of age. He was being penalized because of his honesty and candor in the revelation of unofficial information.

I am yet to see anyone dying or seeking insurance payments for an asymptomatic spinal stenosis. Applicants for insurance coverage must be mindful of the medical history they submit for insurance or any other purposes. Their medical records, although dormant, may return to haunt them for the rest of their lives. Beware of self-diagnosis. Every low back pain does not emanate from degenerative arthritis. Every shooting pain down the leg is not caused by a spinal stenosis, even with a positive x-ray finding. Physicians treat their patients and not the x-ray report. Allow your physician to make the diagnosis. Don't become an unlicensed physician; they are described as quacks in some circles. Your actions may have legal, social, and economic consequences. Many of my senior patients with spinal stenosis are without symptoms. Spinal stenosis does not always indicate the presence of degenerative arthritis; it may occur following a trauma or the result of a congenital defect. I believe that if some insurance carriers have their way, seniors may find it more difficult to be covered.

Long-term insurance is a contract involving the insured and an insurance carrier. The coverage, therefore, will include only those entities or services written in your contract. Your premium payments will be determined by the benefits and the duration of coverage you have contracted to receive. Your insurance policy may cover total or partial cost of nursing home, assisted living, hospice care, day care, adult care, live-in caregiver, and several other benefits. It may also cover a companion or a private duty nurse. Keep in mind, the total cost of benefits would never exceed the policy benefit maximum, although your premium payments may increase. Other factors influencing your premium payments will be the dollar amount you receive per day, whether you are covered at $100, $200, $300, or more each day; the age of the insured, younger insured lower rates; premium are also influenced by the "elimination period."

What is the elimination period? This is the period of paid care before your coverage becomes effective. (You must have paid for your care/treatment for a period of one hundred twenty days before you are eligible to begin your LTC.) It varies according to your contract and may be from zero to as long as 120 days; long elimination period, lower premium payments. Cost of living inclusion is another factor which increases the cost of your long-term coverage.

There is also the possibility that the premium you pay may be eligible for income tax deduction. Benefits paid from your long-term care contract may be excluded from income tax. These and other related benefits should always be verified with your tax consultant since tax laws may change over the life of your contract. For the tax-qualified policy, the insured must qualify and be in need of care for at least ninety days. If the need for care is less than ninety days, this coverage does not come into play. The insured must also be unable to perform two or more activities of daily living (ADL). This ninety-day period is also applicable for any severe cognitive impairment, such as dementia. Benefit payments are usually made directly to the insured who in turn pays the institution or the caregiver. There is the notion that long-term Insurance is for old folks; if this concept implies the inability to transfer from bed to chair or inability to feed oneself independently, then the notion is invalid; I would dispel this notion as being unfounded and without merit.

About 40 percent of long-term care recipients are believed to be between the ages of eighteen and sixty-four. As a resident physician and fellow in physical medicine at Howard Rusk Institute, New York University/Bellevue Hospital, and the Veteran's Administration Hospital, I saw many patients between the ages of eighteen and twenty-eight. These patients eventually required long-term care, following their discharge from acute rehabilitation because of their disabilities and their economic status.

I remember one case assigned to me at Bellevue. It was there I was introduced to the acronym GSW (gunshot wound). I observed with much concern that the common injuries of patients of this age group admitted at the institute/New York University were from diving, trampoline, or automobile accidents and resulted in paralysis at various levels due to spinal cord involvement. The common injuries of patients of this age group (eighteen to twenty-eight) admitted to my service at Bellevue had been gun-shot-wound or leaping from considerable heights. These contrasting etiologies of injuries were very consistent with the socioeconomic environment of the victims, and I felt for these victims of gun-shot-wound a special sense of sadness.

My charge was an eighteen-year-old male who had been shot in the back by the superintendent of a building as he fled from an attempted robbery. This was a very empathic case. His sister had brought him to New York from the South to improve his educational opportunities. He ultimately ended up at a city facility for long-term-care resident at the age of nineteen. This young man was paralyzed in both lower extremities and suffered weakness in both upper, with bladder and bowel involvement. He had failed to acquire a high school certificate; his sister was unable to care for him in her apartment. This was a classic case of a teenager requiring long-term care. My other experience was a thirty-four-year-old college professor who was diagnosed with multiple sclerosis (MS) and required long-term coverage during periods of its exacerbation because of disabling pain and contractures which rendered her wheelchair-bound for long periods during the year. The college professor was covered by long-term care insurance. The eighteen-year-old was eventually covered by Medicaid, a version of long-term care insurance provided by the state and federal governments. Perhaps the most remarkable patient under my care who required long-term care at a relatively early age was a young male who had just celebrated his thirty-fifth birthday when he was diagnosed with multiple myeloma.

The disease process in multiple myeloma invariably invades the skeletal system, much like cancer, causing bone pain, fractures, anemia, and generalized weakness. It may also invade organs, such as the kidneys, causing renal failure. This young man was having a routine x-ray evaluation of the dorsal spine and pelvis because of persistent low back pain and generalized weakness. Following his x-ray, he attempted to get off the table and discovered for the first time that he was unable to move his legs; he had become paralyzed in the lower extremities; his definitive diagnosis was then established. From this time on, he was confined to bed or in a wheelchair. These documented cases should dispel the notion of long-term care being the exclusive domain of "old folks." Long-term care under the circumstances outlined would have provided coverage for these individuals. They were no longer able to perform many of their independent living activities. Coverage in these circumstances may have included care in the home environment, community, or in an assisted living or nursing home facility. Those unable to buy LTI coverage find themselves at the mercy of the Medicaid program. It is estimated that these LTI benefits are expected to cost well over a trillion dollars over the next twenty years. These benefits are significant for the economy:

- They protect the Medicare and Medicaid program.
- They will provide better and enhanced care for seniors and disabled.
- They will provide sustained employment for those who serve as caregivers and related workers.

Once benefit is approved and in effect, your premium payments are suspended for most contracts; this benefit should be written in your contract.

The adverse side of long-term insurance coverage is the frequency with which companies are able to increase the cost of their premiums, with no additional benefits to the insured who has little recourse. These arbitrary increases are the driving forces in the rising cost of health care delivery. Many seniors depend on their long-term insurance to supplement payments for the cost of their assisted or skilled care; although able to live partially independent lives, they require assistance for at least two of their daily living activities, food preparation and baths/showering, which make them eligible for LTI coverage.

Any increase in premium payments will inevitably increase the cost of health care delivery, yet long-term insurance carriers seem to have little compunction in increasing the cost of their premiums. It seems that "the state has no formal ability to approve or disapprove a rate increase upon review of the request of company," according to quotes from one insurance carrier. One insured whom I have interviewed reported that his long-term insurance carrier has notified him in March that an increase in premium of 60 percent is to take effect in May of the same year. The only mitigating aspect in that announcement was that the increase would be phased in over a three-year period, an increase of 20 percent each year. The reason given for the increase was that the expected claims on the carrier, over the life of the insured contract, was significantly higher than what was originally anticipated when the contract was initiated. Would this insurance carrier reimburse the insured if claims were found to be significantly lower than what was originally anticipated? They assured him that the increase was not based on age, health, or claim history; they were based on the judgment of the actuary paid by the insurance company. With a breath of arrogance, the insured was reminded that the contract certificate gave them the right to increase his premium on a class-*wide* basis; they also reserved the right to change premium again in the future if their experience warrants an increase and that it was possible that the premium rate would increase again in the future. You must note that the insurance companies seem to have all the advantages. Premiums always go up; CEOs' bonuses, salaries, and stock options seem to remain intact or increased; the insured seldom, if at all, receive any added benefit.

Long-Term Insurance, a cover for senior care: Savings for elder care during the working period of life has become elusive for most working families of four, two adults and two siblings. Families who prioritize their obligations invariably place insurance for later years, long-term insurance on their back burners. These families will tell you that their first concern is having health coverage for the family. Young working families are not yet eligible for Medicare coverage, and their income not sufficient to allow any meaningful saving program. However, incomes are too high to qualify for any social benefits as Medicaid. This group falls within middle-income America, a rapidly shrinking group, falling just above or at the poverty level; they suffer the most from the health care dilemma we face. The next priority for working families is the educational needs of their children. Although the community colleges play an important role in lowering the cost of education for many residents; families are still expected to make significant contributions toward the education of their sons and daughters, leaving little resources in hand to put aside for long-term care. It takes very skillful financial juggling to balance a budget under these circumstances. For many Middle Americans over the age of sixty, to begin saving for senior care is like "too little, too late," though some may argue, "Where there is a will, there is a way."

Advisors on insurance policies will recommend that LTI begins as early as possible during the working life of an individual. Premium payments are lower when policies are contracted at an early age and more within the financial ability of the insured. A policy for a twenty-two-year-old college graduate would cost a fraction of what one would pay at age sixty. Another advantage often overlooked, the lower premium rate may enable the applicant to negotiate contract for a much larger coverage in benefit. Although these policies serve a useful purpose in later years or during time of disabilities, it must be remembered that LTI are not the usual health care coverage. Being hospitalized may not entitle the holder to any benefits during the period of hospitalization. Benefits must meet specific criteria set by the companies which issue such policies. In general, LTI covers mainly disabilities which are determined by your insurance carrier and are usually specified in your long-term contract. It is important that the insured reads all the fine prints and notes, all the exclusions in the policy, for once the contract is signed, there can be no changes, except for your ever-rising premium payments.

One unpleasant expectation of long-term insurance is their ability to increase their premiums without any corresponding increase in the cost of living or benefits. Budgeting must, therefore, factor these unexpected increments in your planning. I have previously made comments in this book about the financial cost of payments.

The acquisition of long-term insurance coverage or any insurance coverage is a matter for the family to consider and decide. Comments on long-term insurance should not be taken as a disapproval or endorsement of such policies; this is information obtained from observations and the experience of others; they may serve readers only as resources in making informed decisions as to the merit of these and other insurance coverage.

Rising Cost Of Health Care

Every insured and every health care recipient must share some responsibility for the escalating cost of health care. It is a strange paradox that some of the most ardent critics of the system are the largest recipients of the health care largess. On a recent visit to the office of a skin specialist, the doctor was scathing in denouncing the rising cost of health care. He was very critical of two enterprises he singled out as major contributors to this health care dilemma:

- Insurance companies
- Pharmaceutical companies

As I listened attentively, I murmured, "How about the physician? How about the health care recipients?" My experience has already indicted these players. I left he doctor's office with two prescriptions: one for five-hundred-milligram cephalexin capsule, an antibiotic to be taken twice daily; other was for an ointment, bactroban, which incidentally was manufactured in Croatia, to be applied three times daily on the skin. Few people I have asked knew where Croatia was located; this is one of the independent countries which emerged from the breakup of the former Socialist Republic of Yugoslavia in 1991. I was shocked when I got to the pharmacy and inquired about the cost of the ointment which, incidentally, could have been bought over the counter. She advised that my cost was $5. I then asked her what the charges were to the insurance company. She said it would cost them $51.99. I could have purchased a comparable sixteen-milligram ointment for $12.38. Why then does a physician, who was concerned about the cost of health care, prescribe such a costly ointment when alternatives were available at a lower cost? These costs are significant contributors to our health care dilemma. The notion that the cost is covered by private insurance is entirely erroneous. Your insurance carrier may pay for this outlandish charge, but your premium goes up by 29 percent in several months. Who then pays the cost?

One patient who was seen by his surgeon for a follow-up visit which took exactly eighteen minutes of his time, in addition to one blood sample taken by the technician for PSA analysis, was billed for $600. The patient had surgery six years previous and now makes annual follow-up visits; he had no procedures done. When the patient questioned the charges, he was told by the office manager, "Send the bill to your private insurance, they will pay." There was little thought that the patient ultimately must pay for these excessive billings. The bill was sent to the patient's Medicare carrier who showed reasoned judgment and balance and paid less than $100 plus cost of the PSA.

Excessive Prescribing: Many of the prescriptions filled by pharmacies are never used to completion, and this excessive prescribing continues throughout the country. Medicine cabinets in many homes have become veritable drugstores. This practice has no doubt cost tax payers, through their Medicare and Medicaid benefits, billions of dollars over the years. The beneficiaries of such wanton abuse are the pharmaceutical conglomerates and their conduits, the pharmacies, which dispense them and prescribed by physicians who are often unaware of the cost. How does this happen? A patient was prescribed sixty, five-hundred milligram cephalexin to be taken twice daily" for a small infected sebaceous cyst on his back; note there was no time duration in which the medication should be taken. The patient's problem was resolved after a week, but the patient, in his wisdom, continued to take the medication for another week; he had taken a total of twenty-eight five-hundred-milligram capsules; thirty-two capsules were left unused and wasted because medications are nonrefundable and nonreturnable. But for the good judgment and common sense exhibited by this patient, he would have swallowed sixty, 500 mg. cephalexin capsule as prescribed by the specialist/ physician, perhaps to his detriment and most certainly added to the cost of Medicare or Medicaid, with no additional health benefit to the patient. Prescriptions must always be precise as both the pharmacist and the patient rely on the accuracy of the doctor's prescription. Unfortunately, there had been no clear direction by the physician on whom this patient relied for his medical guidance.

Another area for medication waste and cost to the health care system relates to "switch in medications" by physicians after the initial dose was taken by the patient who had been prescribed sixty tablets, taking two tablets daily. It is not uncommon for a physician to change a medication after a few doses were taken by the patient because the medication was found to be ineffective or harmful to the patient. A case in point: Your physician prescribes sixty sixty-milligram unscored tablets to be taken, one tablet at 8:00 a.m. daily after breakfast. However, after taking the first dose, the patient begins to vomit excessively. The physician decides to discontinue this medication or to reduce the strength of the tablets by half. Since unscored tablets cannot be equally divided, the remaining fifty-eight tablets will have to be discarded since medications are not returnable. These occurrences take place daily and at tremendous cost to the health care system. This physician had prescribed the appropriate medication and dosage for the problem presented, but patients may react differently to the same dosage of medication and within the therapeutic range.

"We're all alike, but we're different." Many of these occurrences are beyond the scope of the physician. If one were to scrupulously accede to all the adverse effects of medications listed by the manufacturers, fewer medications would be prescribed. It is the calculated risk we take as physicians for the benefit of our patients; this fact is often not fully appreciated by patients who feel better served by their attorneys than by the dedicated physicians who have just cured their disease.

My only comment on some of the unavoidable events:

- Prescribe fewer tablets/capsule, especially your initial prescription, avoiding the three months' supply.
- Instruct your patients to discontinue medications and contact your office and/or pharmacist in the event of any significant adverse effects relating to the medication.
- Suggest that new patients return for a follow-up visit in several weeks if inclined to do so.
- Make brief notes in patient's charts or records that the patient was thus informed.

There appears to be some hypocrisy in pronouncing strong condemnation of escalating health care cost yet willingly contributing to the cost by indiscriminate prescribing. When unwarranted payments to medical providers are replicated over time, the cost to the health care system is enormous.

Patients and other health care recipients are also willing contributors to this senseless escalation of the health care madness, rising cost. One patient who visits her physician's office regularly was asked, "Why are you always in the doctor's office?" She replied, "Oh! I just want him to check me over since I am in that area. I don't have to pay him anything." This is another misconception which enlarges the dilemma. There is nothing free in the delivery of health care; someone is paying for this unnecessary visit at the other end of the line and rightly resents it. Some insurance carriers seem to pay for whatever statements are submitted for payments with little verification. These incidents are merely the tip of the iceberg and further exacerbate our health care dilemma; they are replicated time and time again during the course of a day at great cost to the system, and there appears to be no end in sight.

It is ironic that a lawmaker, a business executive, with the best insurance and Medicare coverage, walks into the doctor's office at eight thirty in the morning without a scheduled appointment, sees a physician, and his problem happened to be a simple hangover, not requiring a medical visit. My prescription for him would have been "Stay off the bottle." His conduct is dismissed as being unreasonable. The marginal-income full-time worker, on the other hand, who requires food stamps to make ends meet, walks into the doctor's office because she happens to be in the area is regarded as the primary cause of the health care problem. In my view, both actions were unreasonable, reprehensible, and an abuse of the system; they have shown that arrogance of entitlement by their actions and deserved the same condemnation; but one gets a slap on the wrist, the other gets the guillotine. These are the very groups who complain about regulations and regulators. It is as though the robbers are complaining that there are too many cops in the house.

Redundancy in prescribing is another infraction which adds to the coffers of drug manufacturers and unwittingly sanctioned by doctors, patients, and institutions. Patients admitted to institutions are often on several medications; many of these are issued by the local (institution) pharmacist as a "unit dose," with a thirty-day supply on one card. Each tablet or capsule is sealed in its compartment on this card, and the dates are printed aside each compartment, corresponding to the days of the month. This method of dispensing, however, does offer a measure of safety, for if medication was not given to the patient on a given day/date, the pill or capsule would be in its compartment on the following day/date.

The problem arises when the patient is discharged from the institution after spending only seven days, leaving behind thirteen days of prepaid medications on his "unit dose" card. The usual practice when discharged from hospital is to issue several prescriptions for medications patient currently takes each day. One patient received as many as eight prescriptions. Tablets not used were left on patient's card. These new prescriptions are then filled by the local pharmacy, costing hundreds of dollars to Medicare, independent insurers, or co-pay cost to the patient. Your unused medications presumably benefit the institutions or others. Patients have a responsibility to request the return of their prepaid unused medications instead of filling a new prescription for the same medication. A reduction in the number of tablets prescribed may go a long way in mitigating the cost. The cost of drugs is one of the prime movers in the rising cost of health care.

Take the case of a popular drug commonly prescribed for high blood pressure; its patent has long expired, and the generic form is now commonly prescribed. It is now presumed that the original producer of this drug has long recouped the cost involved in its development and marketing.

The federal government in its wisdom has always allowed adequate time, from the initial development of a new drug to the expiration of its patent, for companies to recover their financial outlay and with reasonable profits. These manufacturers have invested considerable sums of money to develop new products, and they deserve adequate returns. This also serves as an incentive for research and development of new products. During this period, the drug is manufactured and sold exclusively under a brand name, the name designated by its original manufacturer. On expiration of its patent, the manufacturer no longer has monopoly, and this drug may then be manufactured and sold by other companies as a generic product. The notion expressed here is a simplistic explanation of a more complex series of events which one may obtain from the Food and Drug Administration, an agency of the U.S. government.

Some institutions and their administrators are complicit in the rising cost of health care by their refusal to accept authentic and identical medications; these were left over due to the transfer of patient from one institution to another. They insist that these medications must be issued by their pharmacies, even at excessive cost to the patients and their insurers who have already paid for these medications. There seem to be a disregard for the cost involved. I have been on the other side of the coin, the physician's side. I now experience the patient's side. The overarching impact of these excesses directly influence the rising cost of health care. Where is the outrage? When I inquired, what happens to the remaining unit dose medications which were not collected by the patient on their discharge, I was informed that they were returned to the pharmacy of the institution which has supplied kit in the first place. My presumption, those medications were not discarded; they were repackaged and resold.

A prescription for generic blood pressure medication was given to a patient, a physician. He was charged $5 by the local pharmacy as his co-payment for thirty 20 mg tablets; this amount, he was told, was set by his insurance carrier. He then inquired about the amount paid by his insurance carrier. He was told that the insurance carrier paid $49.89. The total cost for thirty tablets was about $54.89. The unsuspecting insured thought he had a great bargain, paying only $5. Have no illusion about what was paid by your insurance carrier because that was your money. It came from the premium you and your employer have paid for your insurance coverage each year. My experience has shown that this patient at that time could have obtained the generic medication elsewhere at a significantly lower cost, $3.

The following represent the cost schedule (2012) for one hundred identical generic tablets mentioned:

100, 5 mg. tablets	$6.00
100, 10 mg. tablets	$6.89
100, 20 mg. tablets	$9.89

My patient paid the pharmacy a total of $54.89 for thirty twenty-milligram tablets which cost approximately $3 for thirty tablets when bought through the exchanges known to physicians and other health care professionals. I have no doubt that these exchanges are also making profits, or they would cease to exist. My cost estimate of this generic medication shows that the co-pay of $5 dictated to the pharmacy by the insurance carrier in this context has more than covered the entire cost of the prescription. The vexing question which will remain a secret: "Who keeps $49.89 not accounted for in this transaction?" The patient has already paid more than the entire cost of his prescribed medication with his co-payment. These costs, as I have experienced them, may be described as obscene at best. "Here lies the body of one of our biggest health care dilemma." It will not change until the base causes are identified and accepted as such; then there must be the political willingness to act unequivocally; during this interlude, Middle America continues to suffer the rising cost of health care.

My patient asked me, "Doc, why am I on so many medications? Do I need all of them?" I am sure many physicians are confronted by the same or similar questions. The reflex response is to say yes, but a reflex is a local response and is not mediated through the central nervous system, the brain. A more thoughtful and measured response is to say "Let me review these medications you have been prescribed." This response, however, is a promise which calls for an inordinate amount of time and effort to review the multiplicity of medications this patient had been prescribed by various doctors over time. Your patients are consumers and often feel obligated to ask questions of their doctors, including questions about the medication we prescribe. The avoidance of questions on the part of physicians creates suspicion and a sense of distrust on the part of patients. In the age of the computer and the Internet, our patients are able to evaluate the veracity of physicians about the information we give them. Some patients seem to show better insight about the benefit of medications we prescribe, and those they find ineffective are often added to the list of discarded medications stored in the medicine cabinet; these patients have answered the difficult question we as physicians may be unable or unwilling to answer. Viewed from within, I found some medication prescribed for patients over many years to be ineffective and useless, even by the criteria set by the manufacturers; some eye drops prescribed caused more problems than they resolved; these were discontinued with no adverse effects on the patient and at a savings of hundreds of dollars with each renewal. I have often asked the same question, "Do patients need a prescription for medication every time they visit my office?" The answer is unequivocally no. Some patients have come to believe that a new prescription is an indication of good treatment, a notion which should be strongly discouraged. A few minutes of my time to attempt giving the patient some insight into his problem and the objective of the planned treatment often go a long way toward satisfying the patient's expectation of an office visit.

A word of caution, there may be a down side to those who indiscriminately discontinue their medications without the knowledge or sanction of their physicians; always keep in mind that they are licensed practitioners. Nothing stated here should give you license to be an unlicensed practitioner. The withholding of certain prescribed medications could be life-threatening. One way to avoid overprescribing is to stop new prescriptions for every visit unless there is a very compelling indication. Excessive prescribing by physicians is a tendency which should be addressed. Some patient prescribes, and the doctor writes the order; fortunately, this practice is infrequent but does occur. A young athlete who suffered contusion and strained tendons in his ankle was able to convince his family physician that he needed a wheelchair; whether this was paid for by an insurance carrier or rented by the patient at his expense, the principle of writing a prescription against the better judgment of the physician is being compromised, and the doctor is held in poor esteem by his patient. The wheelchair was never returned to the vendor but eventually stored by this fit and fully mobile individual. All that was required for this patient's mobility was a pair of crutches; although this has not been the rule, it deserves mention as an unnecessary addition to the ever-rising cost in health care delivery. The same is true when sixty capsules of antibiotics are prescribed; the patient takes twenty-eight capsules, his infection has cleared, and he is left with thirty-two capsules to be stored in the kitchen cabinet. Do you continue to drink water after your thirst is satisfied?

Another area frequently abused is in the refunding of dual payments received by doctors and vendors. I have received several reports of patients making co-payments to the vendor or physician who subsequently receives co-payment directly from the insurance carrier. These patients complained that they were not refunded the co-pay made to the vendor. The solution is simply to write to your vendor or physician or a phone call to their office, indicating that you were informed that co-pay was made by your insurance carrier, and your duplicate co-pay would be promptly returned. Another way to avoid this duplication of co-pay is to allow some time to elapse before you make your co-payment. Physicians' offices are usually overwhelmed by paperwork involving patients' records and reports; failure to refund a co-pay check is more likely an oversight than a deliberate attempt to defraud the patient of a few dollars.

CO-PAYMENTS: Co-payments represent a relatively small portion of the patient's obligation, keeping in mind that the patient is always responsible for his medical bills, even though these may be covered by his insurance carrier; in the event your insurance carrier fails to make payment, the patient must assume the responsibility for payments. Co-payment represents the balance due after your carriers have made their payments. Medicare pays up to 80 percent of the amount it approves. The patient or his coinsurers pays the balance. Co-payments may be made either to the patient or to the physician. Some contracts call for co-pay to the physician immediately following his evaluation and/or treatment. The amount is usually fixed by your insurance carrier. You should know that whenever an insurance contract has a deductible option, the patient is responsible for the direct payment of co-pay until the deductible has been satisfied. An annual deductible of $500 mean that the patient is responsible for co-payments totaling this amount during that calendar year. This is another way of increasing your insurance premium during a contract negotiation.

"Insurance premium rocket upward unchecked." It was reported that one insurance carrier had requested premium increase by as much as 24-39 percent. Fortunately, those rates were rejected by state regulators. In one state, increase in premium of 18.5 percent was rejected by the regulators. "In 2009, it was reported that one carrier requested approval of premium increase of 56 percent for some plans." Recent economic data was reported showing profits for ten largest insurance companies increased 250 percent between 2000 and 2009, which was ten times faster than the rate of inflation. The five largest health insurance companies took in profits of $12.2 billion, an increase of 56 percent over previous years. The CEO of these companies were said to have been compensated up to $24 million in 2008. These profits and compensations in the face of the unconscionable increase in premium cost certainly prevent many Americans from acquiring needed insurance coverage. What a dilemma!

Many recipients of health care benefits are totally ignorant of the tremendous cost to the government and ultimately to the tax payers for delivery of health care. Some still refer to the service as "free service." This notion perpetuates the wanton abuse of the health care delivery system by many recipients. Users of the system must be educated in the proper application of health care, and physicians and others must be more scrupulous without denying those in need of health care.

Insurance carriers have been criticized for spending far more than what is considered reasonable for administrative cost. They will spend disproportionately more on CEOs' salaries, stock options, and bonuses than for patients' care. This unbridled and displaced spending has been factors in the evolution of the 80/20 rule in the Affordable Care Act mentioned elsewhere this book. One of the pernicious problems with insurance carriers is their ability to increase their premiums with little or no apparent justification. Often these increases far exceed the annual cost of living. The real problem is the inability of the insured to keep up with the precipitous increase when their wages and salaries remain fixed. Small businesses which contribute to part of employees' insurance coverage also suffer as a result. In spite of these outrageous circumstances, the bonuses, the salaries, the stock options of administrative level personnel have become the "untouchable." To reduce cost of operation means increasing the ratio of care-worker/patient from one to ten, up to one to twelve and to employ more part-time workers with virtually no benefits, impose higher charges for lunches that care workers receive at nominal charges, but never to touch the "untouchable." Unfortunately, these decisions and actions of management always reflect negatively on the quality of care your loved ones receive.

The question frequently asked: What are the criteria for increasing insurance premiums beyond the cost of living index, in the absence of any wage increase for worker, when benefits to the insured remain flat? This is a valid question never answered to one's satisfaction. The insured are often placated by complicated often irrelevant charts and graphs indicating that the amount paid by your insurance carrier exceeds the amount of premium payments received during a given period. But the question which is never answered satisfactorily: "Then why the administrators, the CEO's salary and bonuses are not negatively affected by this calculation?" I do not recall any long-term insurance carrier offering additional benefits other than those written in your contract. Apart from the increments in your premium payments, your benefits are the only part of the equation which remain fixed. It is often overlooked that the increasing cost of health care has a direct relation to increasing cost of premiums paid by the insured or by his employees through payroll deductions.

Many insured are middle-income Americans who are already struggling with other cost-of-living issues of more immediate and urgent demand than the insurance premium due; these include payments for gas and electricity, food, rent, transportation to and from work, and perhaps tuition fees. Some in this income group may include the working poor, "the 47 percent" who work full time at marginal wages and hold a second part-time job just to make ends meet. They are sometimes derided and insulted by politicians and wood-be politicians as being lazy receivers and the like. Their dilemma is that they earn too much to qualify for social programs, Medicaid etc. but not enough to maintain the essentials; some are on fixed income, they receive no cost of living increments; they either lapse in their insurance payments or unable to initiate coverage. The increased premium cost of 8 or 10 percent is more than the prevailing cost of living, and there is no parallel increase in wages or salaries. How are these wage earners expected to cope with such an arbitrary increase?

An important contributor to the health care dilemma is what I have described as "the mathematical absurdity" of the pharmaceutical conglomerates and the insurance monopoly. I also fault users/patients of the system. The fiscal structure of the system could not sustain the spiraling increase in the cost of health care. The absurdity is quite apparent: How can the insured be expected to pay the annual increase of 10-30 percent in premium when he receives only 2 or 3 percent increase in the cost of living? How can the cost of living be frozen at a fixed rate when the cost of health care premium has escalated by 10, 20, 30, and 40 percent? If we accept the headlines in virtually every news publication regarding health care cost, the outlook for the future of health care in America is daunting and dismal. Those who suffer most are Middle Americans who can least afford and often go into bankruptcy, losing their pride and their possessions. Yet there are some defenders of the status quo who are elected to represent the middle-income constituency but being paid by special interest groups to support principles which go against the best interest of the constituency whom they were elected to represent. Where are the gatekeepers and where are those elected to represent our interest? Reasonable Middle America and most consumers accept that in order to thrive, to reward shareholders and executives, and to employ, we must have a profitable and thriving business community, one in which investors and developers of new products prosper. However, when a generic drug is sold to patients for $59.89, which can be purchased at a profit to the agent for $3, then there are questions to be asked about transparency, equity, even morality. Such actions are more perplexing when citizens subjected to these unconscionable price differential are barely living above the poverty line, earning not enough to afford these costs and too much to quality them for Medicaid coverage.

Much credit should be given to the press which relentlessly brings to the attention of the reading public the excesses of unscrupulous executives and their corporations to the chagrin of some executives. These headlines continue to illuminate the front page of publications: "Drug industry seen abuse in discount prices;" these headlines may be laughable when one reads that the drug industrial complex is now complaining of abuse in prices. Sadly, this abuse was always felt by the consuming public. When the drug industry complains about abuse of the health care system, the question then becomes is it because of their compassion or sense of moral outrage that the system and the people it serves are being gouged by heartless benefactors (private oncology practice and community hospital)? Or is it because these groups are getting a bigger slice of the pie than what was anticipated? One only has to review the actual cost of thirty, twenty-milligram hypotensive drug obtained for $3.00, versus what the public must pay through their pharmacies, $54, for the same generic drug. No one should impugn the intent of those responsible for decisions which negatively affects us all; after all, they do give millions on occasion to private institutions, which may indirectly benefit us all, after their stock options, bonuses, and severance settlements are well secured and their names prominently inscribed on buildings. In this captioned article, it seemed that the pharmaceutical conglomerates were incensed that their discount of 20 to 50 percent to agencies that served low-income and uninsured clients were also benefiting Medicare and privately insured patients in addition to the newly formed joint hospital/oncology practice.

It is tempting to conclude that even with the stated discount price of 20 to 30 percent, the drug conglomerates are reaping windfall profits, all from the largess of the government. This supports my prior assertion that the most vociferous critics of the health care system are the largest beneficiaries; it is an interesting paradox.

The conflicting issues in the discount pricing relates to the 340B Drug Discount Program. This drug pricing program was established in 1992 under section 340B of the United States Public Law 102-585 of the Veterans' Health Care Act. This section of the act limits the cost of drugs to federal purchasers and to grantees of federal agencies and to federally qualified health centers (FQHC), disproportionate share hospitals (DSH), and certain groups certified by the U.S. Department of Health and Human Services (HHS). It is said that although the program provided price advantages to low-income groups, the initial participation had been disappointing because the execution of the program was felt to be very complicated for small entities to handle.

The pharmaceutical giants felt that the newly formed joint hospital/oncology practice was reaping large profits by extending the program beyond the agreed entities and at their expense; I doubt that would have driven them into bankruptcy. Those of us who have had experience working in a narcotic addiction program would characterize the entire debacle as a simple case of "drug war," a battle for territorial jurisdiction and price fixing (no pun intended). I shed no tears for the industry. I am convinced that with the enormous profits made by the pharmaceutical industry, the "drug lords" would be economically unscathed. I do empathize with those who must take medications for their health and well-being and pay for the forever-rising cost of drugs.

I have coined the term "mathematical absurdity" to express the disconnect between the escalating cost of health care, the suffering this imposes on middle-income patients and the profits and compensation conjured by the pharmaceutical conglomerate. What is conflicting, although companies declare financial hardship or on the verge of imminent bankruptcy, employees were being furloughed, yet the CEOs and managers continue to receive compensation as though there is business as usual, thus displaying the "mathematical absurdity" here described.

The Swiss citizens, in their effort to bring about transparency, fairness, and equity, seemed to have "tackled the bull by the horn." An independent Swiss politician who had seen the collapse of Swiss International Air Lines in 2001, with rippled effect on his family business, reportedly initiated a nationwide referendum. The objective was to give shareholders of companies listed in the country some influence on executives' and directors' compensation. When a giant Swiss pharmaceutical company decided to pay severance of $78 million to its chairperson, this decision seemed to have generated widespread support for the referendum which, among other restrictions, placed a cap on executive compensation package. These are some of the steps necessary to bring about evidentiary change in the escalating health care cost, but lawmakers must not themselves be the pharmaceutical executives. In evidence of shame and perhaps contrition brought about by the action of a single individual influencing "an educated and committed citizenry," the company reportedly backed off the largess and admitted that "it had been a mistake." It was a mistake only because it was caught and because of the public revolt for such unconscionable and outrageous compensation.

Compensations are said to be voted and awarded by members of the board of directors; most members of boards are recommended by CEOs and the members themselves; they are largely a monolithic group whose thoughts and actions reflect only the philosophy of the board with little regard to any negative impact on the public or the patients they serve. Many believe that these board members/directors are over compensated for the work they perform. The action of the European Union to cap the compensation of CEOs and directors is certainly a step in the right direction in arresting this abysmal trend in executives' compensation which directly influences the rising cost of health care. Some believe that the pharmaceutical industry has done more to increase the cost of health care than any other single entity.

One reads of the antitrust authorities in the United Kingdom accusing a large manufacturer of a brand-name drug of paying off several generic manufacturers to delay the manufacturing and distribution of the generic equivalent into the consumer market. It is reasoned that even after paying large sums of money, amounting to hundreds of millions of dollars, which some may characterize as simple bribery. With all the shenanigan involved, the sick and most vulnerable are left holding the bag while the CEOs are smiling on their way to the bank. It has been estimated that payments to delay the production and marketing of generic drugs have cost American consumers $3.5 billion a year; this is the cost you pay at the pharmacies and through your insurance premiums.

What can the consumer do to prevent or to lower the cost of brand-name prescriptions? Encourage your physician to prescribe the generic equivalent of your medications. Select more OTC medications when you have this option. I have experienced a bill for a "skin protective ointment" prescribed for over a period of three weeks costing close to $108; this ointment has the active ingredient of 99 percent petrolatum which could be purchased OTC for about $15. The same is true for acetylsalacetic acid (Aspirin).

In balance, the public should also know that some generic manufacturers had been deficient in meeting the health codes in their operation in the United States and other countries where they operate. Some have been accused of using substitutes for the active generic ingredients of drugs. Consumers must therefore seek out the reputable generic manufacturers, and there are a number of such companies. Some well-known brand-name manufacturers also make the generic products after the patent has expired.

When enough is enough, public-spirited citizens will come together and speak out in unison, and the watchful eyes of the press will continue to expose. It appears that the pharmaceutical giants take advantage of the most vulnerable and those with the greatest need; to put it into perspective, those whose backs are against the wall.

The philosophy is strictly a business transaction involving supply and demand; you contrive ways to keep the supply low then the demand appears to have increased. A large public demand for a scarce product causes an upward spiral in the cost, even though there is no concomitant increase in the cost of production or marketing. Recent press report has shown the coming together of reputable and distinguished citizens of the world to ask for moral conscience in the pricing of drugs, especially those whose actions destroy malignant cells, cancer drugs.

Evidence for indictment of the pharmaceutical giants for escalating cost continues to be made available by the ever-vigilant press and others. It is sometimes difficult to measure just how much more we pay from month to month and year to year for our medications. For Over The Counter (OTC) medications, the increments are smaller but they occur more frequently during the course of a year. For prescribed medications, especially when covered through your insurance carrier, the annual increase is greater but hardly noticed by the consumer because the co-pay may be as low as $5.00. What is not fully appreciated is that the co-pay is dictated by your insurance carrier, and this is ultimately reflected in the ever-rising cost of insurance premium. Whatever is paid out by the insurance carrier is your collective contributions from premiums paid over time. It is required by law that 80 percent should go toward health care and 20 percent to administrative cost.

A very intriguing way to maintain the high cost of brand-name medications and rising cost of care is by delaying the production and marketing of generic counterpart by smaller drug-manufacturing companies. This is accomplished by paying large sums of money to these smaller manufacturers of generic drugs so that they delay their production and distribution of these drugs at far lower cost, allowing the giants to maintain their reign and dominion over pricing of their already overpriced products. Patients in desperate need of these drugs have experienced cost increase which has more than doubled, although the drug itself has existed for years; there was no cost-of-living increase and no increase in cost of its production or marketing. What then are the factors which influence the increase in cost?

After the cost of cancer drugs had been inordinately increased, costing over $100,000 a year for treatment of one patient, it was time for people of conscience and courage to make their voices heard. An international group of doctors, researchers/scientists, including some who had played important role in the development of the same drugs, took their discontent to the drug manufacturers, expressing their moral outrage over the rising cost of certain drugs desperately needed in the treatment of certain types malignancies. Such expression of outrage by professionals was unique. "Crossing the line of, from essential profits to profiteering" and characterizing drug prices as "astronomical, unsustainable and perhaps even immoral," were expressions seldom used by these respected professionals. In principle, such outrageous pricing on the part of manufacturers is replicated through the industry. When the cost of production and marketing remain stable or flat, the beneficiaries of these increases are largely the companies and their administrators. By their admission, some companies have shown profits in one year to exceed $3 billion when individual patients are virtually going into bankruptcy to pay for the cost of their medical care, primarily for their medications.

Many share the view that with a profit of $2 billion, the distribution of $1 billion to reduce the cost for all patients may have been far more compassionate and appreciative. I am sure that the recipients, whatever they receive, would be appreciative and welcoming, especially when one considers the overall cost each year for most middle-income Americans.

In balance, there is a measure of redemption when large manufacturers of cancer vaccine significantly reduced the cost for poor nations where it was estimated that close to three hundred thousand women lose their lives to cervical cancer each year. Some argue that the cost of these drugs in developing countries, for example India, will inevitably spiral downward because the question of patent, which keeps cost up for these lifesaving drugs, is not sacrosanct. Some countries are known to have disregarded the laws governing patent restrictions and have manufactured similar drugs at a fraction of the cost; their courts have also upheld their rights to do so to save the lives of their citizens. Drug manufacturers in some developing countries are producing these drugs for their domestic use and for export, with impunity and with total disregard for U.S. laws governing their patency. Their actions appear to be fully sanctioned by their judicial system. I presume their rationale, they must do everything possible to save the lives of their citizens, a principle espoused by many life advocates in the United States, even though it means infringement of existing patent. They see saving lives as a moral obligation; few human beings of good will would be against this principle. In some unintended way, we benefit in the United States from many of the low-cost generic drugs manufactured by American conglomerates in developing countries. It is well known that drugs manufactured in the United States are bought at far lower cost in Canada; this is another case of "mathematical absurdity."

MEDICAL IMPLANTS:

Other contributors to the rising cost of health care are the manufacturers and those who implant organs and other medical devices; this group is often overlooked. They are usually higher-income citizens or those well insulated by their affluence. Many of these recipients make independent payments, but for the most part, payments are made through their insurance carriers. These individuals should not be envied for many of them have worked hard, saved long, and able to secure their insurance coverage. At this juncture in their lives, they are certainly entitled to the best coverage they can afford.

In reference to cost, one often hears the expression "Oh! We don't have to worry, our insurance will cover the cost." This flip response, however, overlooks the fact that these individuals are not the sole contributors to the insurance pool from which the cost of their prosthetic hardware and medical/surgical expenses are retrieved to pay at an extraordinary cost. In order to maintain a satisfactory balance sheet, allowing equity for shareholders and bonuses for CEOs, insurance companies justify increasing their premiums which is shared by all insured; this places an untenable burden on those with marginal income who are already struggling to meet their coinsurance payments and other obligations.

A recent recipient of an artificial implant was reported to have remarked, "We have the most expensive health care in the world, but it doesn't necessarily mean it's the best." This reference was made with regard to news coverage comparing the cost of medical implant in the domestic market (U.S.) against implants carried out outside the United States.

Reports have shown that an ordinary hip replacement in the domestic (U.S.) market would cost six times more than it would cost in some European markets. One undergoing these procedures is able to include a European vacation and a follow-up visit. My concern is a shift to the European continent for elective surgical intervention would be like the shift of some of our manufacturing industries; this would not bode well for the delivery of health care in the United States. It is my impression that a source of the problem has to do with the supply and demand for implants and those responsible for their implantation. Another source lies in the number of middlemen involved, from the manufacturing to the implantation of the device, with each intervening functionary receiving a huge slice of the pie.

It is projected the shortage of physicians will become more acute as the population increases and the number of training facilities in the United States unable to close the gap; this imbalance will place an inordinate burden on the supply side of the equation. The relatively few who are skilled and able to carry out these technical procedures find it necessary to charge whatever fees the market would tolerate; keep in mind that fees vary from region to region and from hospital to hospital.

I asked a colleague about the high cost of hip implantation. He was ready to give me a scholarly explanation: "My charges are not unreasonable!" he said. "Don't forget we save lives. We relieve people of their intractable pain and suffering and help them get back to productive work. I have in my office three full-time staff working for me and I carry their insurance. I have retained them whether my income was up or down. I spent innumerable years in college, in professional school, and in training to perfect my skill, foregoing golf and social events most of my friends were able to enjoy and took for granted. Family and social priorities were never met at desirable times.

Life at times became so structured and mundane that this abnormal lifestyle seemed normal and conventional. My work as a professional is always scrutinized for flaws, contrived or real, but which may lead to litigation. This dagger threat is perpetual. For all my travail, I net far less than a million dollar a year."

He continued, "The CEO of my health care system received over ten million in compensation and bonus last year. This was achieved by laying off several hundred hospital and related workers. His organization has rigidly maintained the minimum wage schedule in many of their institutions. Workers have been asked to share a greater part of their health care benefits. Yet they are less often identified as prime cause for the rising cost of health care."

I have not heard an explanation for this difficult issue given with such passion and clarity, which warrants inclusion in this publication.

SALARIES/COMPENSATION: It is generally accepted that there should be reasonable and fair compensation for productive work; such incentive often evokes the best in management and should be encouraged, provided others in and out of the system are not exploited in the process. What then is considered to be reasonable compensation for management? This determination is clearly outside the scope of this publication. However, if compensation to top-level management has risen two hundred times and salaries and wages have remained flat or minimally increased, then there is a problem worthy of remediation.

I have already mentioned in this book the effect of administrative compensation on the rising cost of health care. In this context, it was reported that one health care corporation has seen it fit to progressively increase its executive compensation from five million in 2008 to just over twelve million in 2011. Medicare, Medicaid, and the insured are justified to inquire, "What is the source of such outlandish compensation to CEOs for a single employee?" The simple answer: you, the insured; you, the tax payer; you, the victim of a poorly managed SNF; you, the poorly compensated employee.

It was further reported that admissions had to be suspended at one facility under the umbrella of that administration because of errors in medication, bedsores, and falsified medical records were discovered. Perhaps a smaller compensation may have enabled the institution to add a few more caregivers to reduce the worker-patients ratio and offer better care to the patients they serve.

In reference to CEO's compensation, it was pointed out that CEO pay had little to do with improved performances.

"In fact, some of the country's most highly compensated CEOs over the past decade have presided over huge drop in earnings, loss in shareholder value, massive layoffs, and the underperforming of their workers' pension fund at a time when average workers are experiencing little or no income growth. Many of America's CEOs have lost any sense of shame about grabbing whatever their pliant handpicked corporate board will allow."

Many of the defaults mentioned are directly related to "cutting the corners" and substituting personnel not fully trained or experienced to perform tasks they are assigned. A common default is to substitute a licensed practical nurse (LPN) to perform the task of a registered nurse (RN) which is mandated if the facility is licensed to admit Medicare/ Medicaid patients.

"MEDICATION ERRORS" are serious infractions in skilled nursing facilities and may result in the demise of patients when the incorrect dosage or incorrect medication is administered. It is generally known in the nursing community that bedsores in patients are the reflection of poor nursing care; in fact, it is one of the criteria I used in my quality care assessment table to determine the quality care by an institution.

IMPROPER PRACTICES: The system is also plagued by practitioners who are said to overcharge or charge for services never carried out. Indifference to convictions for fraud meted out by the court, there are those who believe that they can outsmart the system. A recent allegation by the federal government, one practitioner in a four-year period had performed twenty or more operations in a course of the day and treated, on average, sixty patients is a case in point. During the same period, it was alleged that this practitioner had submitted claims in excess of $30 million to insurance carriers.

The transgressors also include those who sell controlled substances at enormous price, often without seeing the patient. These operators simply write prescriptions, a very dangerous practice which endangers the health of the victims and increases the cost of health care for those covered by Medicare/Medicaid or privately insured; the premium for the insured eventually goes up. No one wins because the practitioner, sooner or later, is convicted, and the victims are left to suffer with their addiction.

One colleague expressed his displeasure by challenging a bill he had received for $600 for a fifteen-minute follow-up office visit. The billing service was unaware that he was fully conversant with Medicare requirements regarding charges and time spent for office visits. Medicare has specified the amount of time and charges for various visits. An initial consultation should require about forty-five minutes or more according to the intensity of the evaluation; for follow-up visits, the examination is less intense, less time utilized, and cost less. Charges and fees allowed vary according to specialty and location. The charges allowed at large metropolitan cities, especially the large medical centers, do not prevail at smaller suburban clinics and hospitals. Medicare intervened for my colleague, and the problem was resolved to the satisfaction of all concerned. Unfortunately, there are those who are bent on defrauding the system and will continue with such practice.

The single-minded drive to make money at any cost has driven some practitioners to be engaged in events and practices which are clearly beyond the pale. The frequency of their actions had been so routine and traditional that they have become a culture. I refer here to doctors who have "joined in matrimony" with drug manufacturers and producers of surgical devices and implants to virtually deprive insurance carriers and those for whom these appliances are prescribed.

How are these practices carried out? These practitioners, not uncommonly department heads and chiefs of services, also receive payments with the understanding that they would only prescribe products manufactured or produced by the company with which they have a salaried contract. By virtue of their positions, they are able to exert influence, sometimes pressure, on the department as a whole to use only products which they recommend. This philosophy "it is my opinion, therefore our belief" bodes poorly for those who are compelled to use these medications and appliances because their recommendations for alternatives are denied. In some cases, those products compared poorly in quality with others sold in the open market, yet they are sold at higher cost to their coerced and entrapped users by unscrupulous leaders in the profession. Greed and selfishness seem to overwhelm the conscience and humanity of these souls for the extra dollars they can well afford to do without.

Clearly, increase to the cost of health care by unscrupulous operators has little to do with the adequacy or inadequacy of funding but everything to do with those traits listed here and those without scruples; these operators are bent on extracting from the system every resource possible and by any means. Paradoxically, they represent the honest broker, the department head, and the very ones who vehemently complain about the rising cost of health care and who despise recipients of Medicaid. The reference takes on the usual cliché, "those and them."

The dilemma we face: How can the cost of health care be contained when those trusted with the task of resolving the problem are found to be the most intransigent contributors to the problem?

THE IMMIGRANTS'
CONTRIBUTION

We now know that the immigrants' contribution to health care in relation to the proportion withdrawn had been significant. The common belief that immigrants had been a drain on the health care system is now debunked. When events go wrong and sponsors lack the integrity to accept responsibility, there is always the proclivity to look for scapegoat, the immigrant population. The undocumented immigrant has been the convenient object, the scapegoat. Employers take full advantage of their status and their skills; they are paid the lowest wages; health and other benefits are neglected. Whatever tax contributions and other payments made on their behalf are never retrieved for fear of retribution. We now know that the immigrant population has paid more than their fair share into the health care system from which they neglect to withdraw.

When you hear the wailing warning *siren* of a fire truck at two o'clock in the morning, you instinctively get out of bed; some occupants will rush to the exit door or window and look in the direction of the wailing sound of the siren. For that moment, you are unaware that the firemen are responding to smoke gusting through the partially opened window of your kitchen on the first floor. Your house is on fire, the kitchen is being engulfed by the inferno while your tunneled vision is focused on the street and the neighbors next door. You must have concluded that "There is a fire on the block, but it could not be our home. You were quite wrong, and this denial cost them their home.

There was the implied belief that the bad events would not befall them. This narrative has brought into focus the first positive development in the rising cost of health care and published in *Health Affairs*. There is the tendency to look toward others for problems we create. The thought that someone else is responsible for our ill-fated adventures seems to relieve us of the responsibility we are unable or unwilling to confront or to accept and resolve; because of this convoluted reasoning, we repeat the same mistakes, create the same problems, and continue to blame others when we should be thanking them for their benevolence.

Immigrants were often singled out and maligned as among the prime causes of our heath care dilemma; this group is often accused of being a burden to the various local and state health clinics. "They come without insurance. They overburden our school system." The negatives are unrelenting and sometimes acrid. Yet the immigrant workers continue to toil in their respective occupations, filling the vacuum in our workforce created by the refusal of the American workers to work the twelve and sixteen hours' day, yet live at the poverty level; these and other contributions which the immigrant workers provide are ignored by their critics who only see these workers as "those people who crowd our hospital clinics and take away our jobs." It is sometimes a case of "the dog and the manger."

At last, the day of redemption has come for the undocumented immigrant worker with the findings of research studies from reputable institutions as Harvard University and the City University of New

York. This group has conducted studies on immigration reform, and the findings were startling. The study shows that the immigrants are subsidizing Medicare instead of draining it.

Immigrants have contributed to the Medicare Hospital Trust Fund and account for almost half of Medicare revenues and that pays for hospital care in excess of their use of it. The surpluses totaled $115 billion from 2002 to 2009. It further showed that American-born populations had a deficit of $28 billion over the same seven-year period. The Harvard/CUNY study shows that immigrants are paying billions of dollars each year, much more than they use in the health care they receive. In fact, the immigrants are subsidizing Medicare by billions of dollars each year. This subsidy is paid each year into the Hospital Insurance Trust Fund. This fund pays for the Medicare part A, which pays for such services as inpatient hospital care, skilled nursing care, home health care for seniors and disabled. For the year 2012, it is said that the Medicare trust fund has assets of over two hundred twenty-five billion. American-born citizens are said to receive about twenty-nine billion more than they contribute to the system. Although the figures used here are not precisely those of the study group, they offer a good source for prediction of current and future trends in the health care dilemma.

I believe the relatively large contribution to the system by the undocumented immigrants lies in the fact that many of these workers abstain from visiting clinics or emergency rooms out of fear of deportation, yet contributions to the system have been made by their employers. I have treated one undocumented worker for several months without any compensation; this gentleman was injured at his workplace, at a construction job. He had suffered compressed fractures in the lower spine with weakness in both lower extremities and unable to walk independently. It was a pathetic situation; this young construction worker was never covered by any insurance as his American colleagues were covered. The owner/contractor tried to relegate this employee as an independent contractor to avoid paying insurance premium or taxes on his behalf; the poor guy hardly spoke English. His English was such that his medical and related history were obtained through an interpreter. His colleagues, workers from his native home, visited often, and they all attested that he was the best worker. He had perfected his trade as a brick layer and builder in his native country. This worker was certainly an asset to his employer, a good worker being paid $15 an hour working long hours and on weekends, including Sundays while his boss prayed for his mercy. He received no other benefits, except being picked up in the morning and dropped off in the evenings. He was "the goose that laid the golden eggs." I was never able to talk to his employer who was said to have visited only twice during the extended hospitalization of his trusted worker. His visits were always at nights; it was so characteristic that I jokingly referred to them as his nocturne in A minor.

I have chosen to highlight these contributions of the undocumented immigrants because these are always buried in the sand. The problem, as I view it from within, is not the undocumented immigrant as some proclaim. The problem lies in the hands of the citizen contractors who enrich themselves on the backs of the immigrant workers whose services and labor are preferred above those of American citizens, including our veterans who are desperately searching for a day's work. Fifteen dollars an hour with full benefits may have been welcomed by a youngster looking for his/her first regular employment.

I have long maintained and confirmed by my experience that our inability to contain the escalating health care cost also relates to the knee-jerk reaction to invent scapegoats as a diversionary alternative for the real problem. The undocumented immigrant population is presently the scapegoat and used effectively by some lawmakers. The notion has found a gullible and receptive following in segments of the population where unemployment is high and many citizens are without health care coverage. We place the blame for our ills on the weakest among us, those who are too timid to refute these absurdities for fear of exposing themselves to the authorities and subjected to deportation. The studies here mentioned will serve to counter some of the allegations that the immigrant workers are the sources of all of our health care problems in relation to cost and if we get rid of them, we will solve the problem of rising cost. This is a simplistic view unworthy of any rationality.

The bigger question: "How could this undocumented worker without any credentials, who was being paid directly by the company, be an independent contractor?" I am still trying to ascertain. It was heartrending to see the number of professionals, orthopedists and physiatrists who participated in the care of this young man knowing that there was no financial gain in assuming care of this human being. The medical profession, as a whole, is sometimes negatively stereotyped when the accusing finger should be pointed only to a few bad apples. With these revelations of contributions of the immigrant workers into the health care system and receiving relatively little in return, the paranoia that immigrants are the cause of our health care dilemma is debunked.

One of the saddest cases in my experience was that of an immigrant worker whose status was undetermined. By his admission, he lived in the United States for nearly a decade but spoke virtually no English. He worked as a dishwasher at a diner, making minimum wages. I had doubts that he had any insurance coverage from his employers. He was referred to me to assist in clearing a storeroom. He was hardly able to speak, not because of language barrier but because of an apparent upper respiratory infection associated with an allergy. He told me he felt hot; he had a fever but insisted that he wanted to help. A simple visit to a doctor or the emergency room would have solved his problem. I suggested that he visit his doctor for treatment or go to the emergency room.

It transpired that this young man had no money to go to a private doctor and was afraid to go to the hospital emergency room. It appears that dishwashers do not do as well as waiters because they do not collect tips. His wages barely sustained him from payday to payday and had no insurance. I was moved to unload professional samples I had obtained and provided some funds for him to go home and remain home for several days. His immigration status was of little concern to me as his medical needs overwhelmed that consideration. To be employed and without insurance coverage or to be desperately afraid of visiting a hospital emergency room for needed treatment are situations which one would only fully appreciate by having the personal experience. There may be countless such immigrants in the cities and towns of this nation. They are not all undocumented, but they are all afraid.

I would suggest that the prime cause of the rising health care cost is within the system itself. It continues to elude those who are elected to resolve the problem because they are looking beyond the contributors of the problem, who are within the system; instead, they are focusing on the least likely group, the undocumented immigrant population. The studies have shown that whatever this group gets out of the system is minimal and insignificant.

The Advocate

The interest of those infirmed and confined to institutions requires regular oversight, someone who will be their mouthpiece to ensure that their care is of the highest quality as required by law. Their needs are best served when there are *advocates* and *advocates* outside the control of the institutions; these may be family members, friends, or independent authorized agencies.

When I inquired at one of the SNFs about patient's *advocate*, I was told that "Every member of my care services is a patient's advocate." This is a glorious expectation, but in practice, it does not occur. It is similar to how a Caribbean friend described his government as: "Hold me shove me,' no advocacy, a state of inertia.

One nurse advocate who was in charge of this unit insisted on discontinuing the weekly shower for one of my patients, explaining that the patient was too weak to sit in the shower chair. I was left without words at this suggestion by this nurse/advocate. I asked her, "How is it that the patient is able to sit in a wheelchair all day but cannot sit in a shower wheelchair for half an hour?" She was obviously embarrassed by her explanation and offered no reason, except that it was less work for the staff. As it transpired, this nurse was yielding to the wishes of one of the aides who found it more convenient to give the patient a so called bed bath than a weekly shower preferred by the patient. Incidentally, this patient was paying $15,000 each month for her SNC. Such was the advocacy of "every member of my care staff."

Social services have always exercised the role of patient's advocate. In credit to this service, it has always tried to bridge the "no man's land" between patients and those who administer and those who give care. "An advocate is one who pleads for a cause or a purpose." In the case of SNF, the cause is the patient, whose disappointments, frustrations, dissatisfactions are sometimes overwhelming. The function of social service, always an agent of the institution, ceases to be absolutely objective. The social worker, as the designated patient's advocate, is a paid employee of the institution and, as such, may wish to exercise the utmost of restraint in representing the rights or entitlements of the client/patient. "You never bite the hand that feeds you." This notion that all workers in a skilled care facility are patient's advocate is, therefore, a utopia. However, the notion, if implemented, would advance the care of the sick and disabled beyond our imagination. Our best advocates are caring members of the family and friends, especially those with some medical/nursing knowledge or understanding. Another advocate may be your family physician and your clergy.

I recall my experience at a major teaching hospital, I insisted that the arm of my CVA patient be kept in abduction using a pillow.

The nurse in-charge grew tired of my insistence and said to me, "Dr. Estwick! If I were a CVA patient, I would want you to be my attending physician." After a pause, she deflated my ego and added, "But I sure hate working for you." The input of the social worker as an advocate may also be clouded by his/her personal bias.

I caution that there is a fine line between those whose intent and actions may be characterized as troublemaking and a humbug and those who are sincere and dedicated advocates. Beware of those who exploit real problems and concerns of patients for the sole purpose of serving their financial and social objectives. I have seen an "advocate" visiting a patient only after it was mentioned in course of a social conversation that the patient had slid out of his bed which had only the upper half of the rail in place. He showed more concern about the height of the bed and enquired were there pads on the floor, how helpful were staff members, did they send him for an x-ray? Clearly, these questions would not serve the immediate need of the client/patient. I would have been more impressed by questions relating to injuries and immediate actions taken to address these injuries and any sufferings. There were no questions about the patient himself, only about the circumstances of the incident. In general, advocates are concerned about patients, the timely administration of therapy and medications, prompt and regular changes for the incontinent patients, safe environment, timely assist in feeding, baths, toilet, and in their recreational needs.

PHYSICIAN/ADVOCATE: My inside view as an advocate and a rehabilitation specialist has allowed me to experience many unique health care adventures. I was exposed to statements, interventions, and decision making best described as phantasies. One incident which still stands out is that of a seizure patient on a standard and well-known antiseizure medication. As the medication accumulates in the system in excess of the therapeutic level, there is a tendency for some patient to react. A common reaction is skin rash, especially over the exposed parts of the body: the arms and forearms, the lower neck, the upper chest. This drug also has a tendency to accumulate in the cortex for long periods; other problems are sedation, unsteady gait, difficulty in swallowing; the drug has also been associated with excessive growth of the gum (hypertrophy) in some people. After I saw this patient scratching the arms intensely, I was drawn to observing more closely. My observation revealed extensive areas of rash over the upper chest and both arms and forearms.

Being aware of the chain in administrative command and my respect for the system of operation at the institution, I called the attention of the LPN and requested that she alert the attending MD so that he may examine the patient on his next ward round. The LPN came to the patient's room with an associate, another LPN, looked at the patient's arm, and said, "Oh! That's not a rash, that's goose pimples. It's cold in this room," which she did not address. It may have been cold from the air-conditioner in the patient's room, but this advocate knew the clinical difference between goose pimples and skin rash. Subsequent blood test confirmed that the drug level was well above the recommended dose that the medication was immediately discontinued. This LPN always had an answer, the wrong one.

When an individual is removed from the cold environment and placed in a warm environment, goose pimples will usually disappear. To my dismay, this LPN had never made notes of my complaint nor did she report it to the attending MD. The so-called goose pimples had not left the patient in over three weeks, the longest continuous goose pimples I had seen in my entire career. This skin rash, incidentally, was an early indication that the blood level of the medication had exceeded its therapeutic level.

One night, about nine thirty, I received an urgent call from the nurse in charge. I first felt that perhaps it was about the demise of the patient for whom I had been the advocate. I was relieved that this was not the case, but the physician on call had ordered an immediate hospital admission for the patient. I asked, "What was the reason for this urgent referral to the hospital?" The nurse related that the blood level of the medication was very high. I was satisfied that the level given me could be lowered without resorting to an emergency hospital admission. I inquired about vital signs and other relevant information. I then told the nurse, "Please do not send this patient to the hospital miles away and at 10:00 p.m. for a high blood level of a medication which existed during the day." I told her to stop the medication, give fluids as permitted, and alert the regular attending physician. This patient was seen by the regular attending physician on the following day, and in a very calm and confident manner, he decided to keep the patient in the unit and followed the "watchful waiting" principle of the seasoned confident physicians of the old days; he also ordered a follow-up blood evaluation. This level of "micromanagement" had prevented a hospital admission which was later determined to be a non-emergency. The patient was relieved of a needless traumatic disruption. The tremendous cost to the health care system was avoided.

Another patient for whom I had advocacy was transported to the hospital from a skilled nursing facility a period of one week for what was described as "altered mental status." This diagnosis gives little information and usually made by the staff and concurred by some physicians who are not inclined to make a hospital visit or those without a clue as to what is happening with their patient. It is a diagnosis that impresses no one in academic medicine, sometimes reflecting negatively on the physician when this is seen as a pattern. Uprooting your senior patients from their usual and familiar domicile, whether to a hospital or elsewhere, is one of the more disquieting and mentally traumatic events these seniors could experience, especially when carried out for a contrived emergency admission or for the convenience of the staff.

Advocate: Not infrequently this practice is carried out only because of convenience or lack of experience of the physician who prefers to err on the side of caution rather than risk the possibility of malpractice and liability; these individuals do well as research scientists where risk-taking and liabilities hardly exists. I have always lectured to junior house staff that physicians must be physicians and never abdicate their clinical judgment and responsibilities to the nurse in charge; you are less likely to be respected by the very staff members, who see such action as a dereliction of duty. Ultimately, your patients and their family-advocate will join the chorus and question your competence as a physician.

Serving as advocate for my spouse had been a unique experience. A limited review of the literature failed to show advocates who were both physicians and spouse, "spousal physician advocates." My role in this unique capacity has given me insight in the mechanics of care, especially skilled nursing care (SNC). As a rehabilitation specialist, I was fully aware of many of the expectations and limitations in medical management. I hasten to mention that some of my judgment in this capacity may have been blunted in its objectivity. Hence, much caution and forbearance were exercised to avoid the often used cliché of "micromanagement"; this is sometimes used by physicians as a tool to discourage any oversight and to cover shortfall (misstep).

Physician/Advocate: I have recommended that clients/patients, especially those spending much of their days in the wheelchair or in bed, should be checked at least every two to three hours during the day. This routine avoids consequences of intolerable odor of urine and feces, skin irritation, maceration or infection, and, worst of these, avoiding urinary tract infection (UTI). This is usually an ascending tract infection and the result of fecal contamination allowed to remain in place for extended time. I have seen this occurring in patients who have been made to endure this intolerable and dehumanizing experience for four long hours. To express my dissatisfaction, I have pointedly asked one caregiver, "Would you personally tolerate such a state of deprivation for four hours without being cleaned?" She declined an answer. Bed baths are usually done for the convenience of staff, but wheel-chaired patients and those able to sit in chairs deserve showers at regular intervals.

A case in point: Your loved one spiking a temperature, origin unknown, is cause for your concern, especially when this is going on for several days, and Tylenol is being given by the LPN to lower the temperature with little success. The day is Friday. The MD would not be in until Monday. It is very tempting in this scenario to ask: Would the nurse take a catheterized specimen of urine (CSU)." Or contact your MD because this looks like a urinary tract infection (UTI), which calls for immediate treatment. Ultimately, this was ordered by the attending MD, and UTI was in fact confirmed, and treatment was prescribed.

I am convinced that this advocacy was in the best interest of the patient. The advocate was well qualified and experienced, but with all the good intent, it may have been perceived as "micromanaging." It is the kind of intervention the advocate without medical experience must tread cautiously; physicians do not take this kindly, even though the patient benefits. This is the kind of dogma in many of us which should be expunged. It is not about us; it is about the health and well-being of our patients. Perhaps the solution is to place ourselves as physicians at the other side of the coin; we may see things quite differently as I have been privileged to see.

Micromanagement: I was never intimidated by this characterization and on occasion, I have used the term but with some regret. I now fully recognize and understand its genesis when it is used by professional colleagues. What was tooted as micromanagement saved me from an unnecessary litigation because of an omission in my management. I quickly became aware that even specialists could benefit from their perception of micromanagement. We cannot be expected to know everything, even within the realm of our specialties except perhaps in the eyes of the trial lawyers, then we wished we were micromanaged. I urge that physicians use micromanagement to their advantage. It is one of the necessary thorns in medical practice which has kept us on track, even though we may deny this; it is here to stay. "Is there a place for micromanagement?"

To give a balanced view, another perspective to the principle of micromanagement is presented. When you elect or agree to have a physician care for your loved one, it is assumed that you were aware of his/her qualifications and to some extent, his ability as a physician; this implied agreement places the patient under the exclusive medical control of this attending physician or his associates.

A physician cannot be expected to be held responsible when an intruder tries to manage. There cannot be two captains in control of one ship. Unless this philosophy is accepted, it is time to get someone else to manage the care of your loved one. Your attending is no longer an intern physician. The human side of this dilemma makes it difficult to accept the concept of micromanagement in spite of what may be perceived as advantages. "Is there a place for micromanagement?" This author has expressed some reservation about the application of micromanagement when not prudently and discreetly applied.

Family Advocate: Spouses and some immediate family members with Power Of Attorney have served as advocates for their loved ones. This practice should be encouraged as it provides another level of oversight. It is well known that whenever a staff becomes aware of the interest and concern of the family, especially those who visit often, your loved ones receive a somewhat higher level of care. Interest and concern do not imply getting in the way of routine staff intervention and care or a complaint for every imagined or real shortfall in the care of a family member. There is a human component to care, and in my experience, there is no perfect care; it is often a matter of give and take. Areas of common concerns for family advocates are usually personal hygiene care, dietary concerns, and social interactions. Question often raised: "Are the toilet needs of the patient attended at regular intervals, especially in those patients who may be incontinent or otherwise unable to relate to staff that they have to be toileted?" Frequent toileting by staff is always a source of contention because the process is cumbersome and the staff would rather avoid this if they are not well supervised.

Unlike the social worker, the family as advocates would not be afraid or intimidated to confront if necessary, the administration on behalf of his/her loved ones. Advocates also must exercise utmost respect and good judgment in deference to care workers, staff, and administrators who are generally doing their best for the clients/patients they have the privilege to serve. Advocates with training and experience unique to the patient's problems must also exercise extreme prudence; they should avoid direct intervention when the staff takes a course of action believed to be contrary to the usual practice or fails to take one, unless the safety of the patient is placed at eminent risk.

I urge the family to continue their advocacy but be respectful and mindful of the effort and the dedication of physicians and care workers. You must call the attention of the physician or the care worker to the rash on your loved one's chest and arms which has gotten worse in several days. You should enquire whether your loved one had a shower in several weeks. You should inquire about the small blister on your loved one's heel. In a bed-bound relative, you have to ask the supervising nurse whether an air mattress may be useful in preventing bedsores.

You do not have to be a physician to ask these questions. Some of these occurrences may escape, even the most observant and dedicated physician. Some institutions may quibble to provide mattress which prevents bedsores, but such preventive measures should be the responsibility of the institution. Institutions have been held liable when patients under their watch have developed bedsores; these are usually attributed to poor nursing care. SNFs must provide an environment which precludes the occurrence of these preventable health issues. Patients and their loved ones ought not to be expected to make special payments for such preventive care appliances; the alternative is frequent mobilization of clients by staff required by state, which may prove to be more costly to institutions in labor and liability.

Skin care, podiatric care and oral hygne: These are areas often overlooked by both caregivers and advocates; they must be included in your concern about the care your loved ones receive. Omission of care in these areas, however, may be the result of oversight by caregivers rather than willful neglect and should be dealt with very discreetly by advocates. In relation to dietary needs, regular fluid intake, especially in the summer months, should be a concern. Dehydration affecting children and seniors is a common occurrence, sometimes resulting in the demise of seniors. The best treatment for this is prevention. Access to water and appropriate beverages is very desirable so that these may be offered to your loved ones ad.lib. So far as nutrition is concerned, I would recommend an appointment and a short visit with the dietitian who is usually willing and able to offer concise and pertinent information to answer your concerns. The integration of food to fulfill the appropriate dietary need is a separate area in medical management about which many physicians, nurses, and care workers are less informed. In practice, I consult our dietary specialists, informing them of the special needs of patients; they in turn will conceptualize the appropriate diet to meet those specified needs. Dietitians are specialists in their own rights; they are trained and certified by state agencies. Their services in management of senior patients should be more widely utilized than is currently being practiced. They do have an important place in medical management and rehabilitation.

Activities: There are few substitutes for the various recreational activities offered to seniors in a skilled nursing facility. Activities such as music, poetry reading, and other suitable scripts of interest, to outdoor games, puzzles involving the hands, suitable movies and visitation are useful. Beware that in many activities, there may be little or no perceived active participation by clients/patient; this, however, should not disqualify patients from inclusion in these activities. It has been observed that many patients receive more sensory/motor stimulation from some of these activities than is usually perceived. The closure of participants' eyes during some events is no indication of the level of their reception; patients left alone in isolation in their rooms is not an acceptable alternative.

Skilled Nursing Facility (SNF)

In earlier years, the term used to described a skilled nursing facility was simply nursing home; this seemed to have accurately described the function of these institutions. People in their later years or those unable to care for themselves were housed and their various needs were served as best as the individual home was able to provide.

Skilled nursing facilities are also referred to as long-term care facilities, are licensed by the various states' Department of Health, and required to meet certain standards set by the federal and state governments to be eligible for Medicare and Medicaid reimbursement. They must also provide adequate licensed support staff coverage to provide for skilled nursing and activities of daily living (ADL) twenty-four hours a day; they must also be under the direction of a licensed physician. A licensed physician should also be available or on call in the event of any medical emergency. Proper records of all medical interventions must be safely maintained and available for inspection by authorized people.

It is recommended that anyone seeking residency in a skilled nursing facility should obtain information from the facility itself, from the state Department of Health, or from the federal Department of Health and Social Services. A visit to the facility and informal talks with staff and family of patients are helpful in order to form a balanced impression of the institution. I have found that printed brochures and commercial ads do not always present the full picture. I have seen brochures with glowing photographs of African Americans and Latinos as residents; in fact their has not been any in residency at the facilities to the memory of the staff working there for over a decade; these groups generally worked as caregivers, housekeeping, and lower-level nursing care. The objective of these ads may be to encourage minority groups to apply for residency and may not imply any deliberate deception.

My view from within has left me with the sad and regrettable conclusion that a number of SNFs, especially those charging higher fees for occupancy, exercise policies akin to being discriminatory. They are more likely to reject applicants in dire need of skilled nursing care. Imagine a skilled nursing care facility refusing skilled nursing patients because there is too much SN involved in their care, a strange paradox indeed. They show preference for those applicants who require custodial care and management or assisted care, to the exclusion of those in need of skilled nursing. I suspect that the task and the responsibility of skilled nursing are too arduous and exacting for administrators and staff of many of these skilled nursing facilities, some of which are operated by business CEOs with Wall Street orientation rather than by people who are also trained and experienced in medical administration. Have no illusion, it is a business operation, but there should be some human component; we are not dealing with inanimate objects.

One applicant with history of post-stroke seizure disorder controlled by medication but required some monitoring was flatly rejected for admission by the CEO. This applicant was tentatively approved by the nursing manager who had evaluated the candidate in person. *I* was appalled by the reason stated for the rejection of this candidate. It reminded me of one of my novice supervisors ignorant of the facts, unprepared and unable to offer a plausible reason for her administrative decision. She wrote, "Given the acuity of our current patient population, we cannot deliver the amount of care the patient would require without compromise to other patients' care needs." I am still struggling to understand what was meant by "acuity of population." This statement by the CEO, in her wisdom, added noting substantive to her reason for rejection of a well-suited and deserving candidate; my reviewer dismissed this reply as verbiage. These events have firmly supported my belief that many SNFs are unable or unwilling to cope with any nursing challenges when these relate to skilled nursing of their charges; they prefer to do what they do best, custodial care. They are reluctant to take patients requiring intravenous administration, regular injections, feeding tubes, wound care, TPR monitoring, and SNC needs.

At another facility, one applicant for subacute rehabilitation who was recovering from a stroke was rejected for admission; the reason given, "there was no bed available." As a consultant at that facility, I knew this was not the case, and I pointedly challenged the director of social services. By the end of that day, the patient was offered a bed and was admitted for subacute rehabilitation on the following day. Under these strange circumstances, one is not paranoid to perceive certain discriminatory practices which have nothing to do with the patient's medical history and eligibility. When an applicant with adequate funding and appropriate medical needs is rejected before submitting all of the required documents, think a second time; the rejection may have some sinister connotation. These intrigues have created a health care dilemma for many applicants, especially those of middle income and below this margin. Many of these patients are hurried out of the acute care hospitals because their acute medical problems have been resolved. Their medical problems are still too complex to be cared for in their homes, yet they are turned down by the SNF with meaningless statements: "Given the acuity of our current patient population," whatever is implied by this statement. Skilled nursing care not only implies skilled personnel but also conditions and equipment necessary to execute such care. Mattresses and the like to prevent the onset of debilitating conditions as bedsores are, therefore, common to these institutions.

THE STROKE PATIENT: Care of the stroke patient and others confined to wheelchairs at some SNFs seemed to be placed into the status of "benign neglect" with regard to prevention of contractures and other flexion deformities. The term was coined by the late Daniel Patrick Moynihan in 1970, when, as the urban affair counselor to President Nixon, he was said to have written a memo:

> "The time may have come when the issue of race could benefit from a period of benign neglect, a period in which Negro progress continued and racial rhetoric faded."

This view seemed tantamount to the expressions "watchful waiting" or "hold me shove me" used elsewhere in this book. It means do nothing, and this is not helpful to those in desperate need and seek our help and expertise.

Many infractions noted in care could be averted if there were proper supervision and training. In the previous section of this book, I have written in some detail about notable deformities occurring in victims of a stroke, especially those confined to wheelchair, unable to walk. Stroke patients with predilection to develop contractures are more likely to suffer from the omission of certain basic preventative care, which could be given by most caregivers; they require little time to execute with training and supervision. Immobility from any cause will result in restrictions at joints and weakness of muscles,

175

but the kind of restrictions noted in victims of stroke is unique. The movements observed in the affected extremities of the stroke victim are essentially reflex in origin. They are not willed movements. Hence, they are more difficult to control. Medications and related procedures which offer some relief of these movements are outside the scope of this book. Suffice to mention that there are hopes for these patients when conventional modalities fail.

It was of interest to note that nearly all facilities offered some form of movement exercises for those who were functional and able to walk—some with assistance, others without. These programs were desirable and no doubt, prolonged the mobility of those who participated; they maintained and improved their ADL functions and their psychological well-being. Similar programs for wheel-chaired patients were notably lacking. There seems to be a different mind-set for those who are relegated to wheelchairs, regardless of the reason for their confinement. I found this practice to be discriminatory and unacceptable. The stroke victim seemed to bear the brunt of this "benign neglect." Every sedentary patient/client may benefit from some form of movement exercise.

To resolve the problems of movement exercise for SNF resident, there must first be the recognition that a problem exists; instead, one sees the characteristic "knee-jerk" response of denial. Clearly, the intent of management is never to cause harm to their clients/patients, but the lack of awareness by administrators and supervisors results in preventable disabilities in a number of wheel-chaired residents at many SNFs. There is the assumption that all residents in wheelchairs are mentally challenged in some manner. It is important that all caregivers rid themselves of such belief; there is the instinctive tendency to treat these residents as such. Similar thought process is in operation for those residents who suffer from expressive/motor aphasia (inability to verbalize). Regrettably, many caregivers lack the understanding of many of the fundamental problems affecting their charges and are unable to deal with them when they occur.

Wheelchair Activities: Physical/functional activities for wheel-chaired residents are as important to them as the activities provided for those with mobility. Wheel-chaired residents especially those who are able to maintain self-feeding, oral hygiene, facial care, ability to turn in bed, ability to extend their heads, and observe a television program or to accommodate the prescribed eye-drops are cost effective to SNFs. The cost to the institution of feeding and oral care of one resident is significant. Perhaps the bigger gratification is the feeling of independence and well-being these functions give to the resident. One patient who came to my attention was an eighty-year-old male who suffered a stroke and had completed his post-stroke rehabilitation. This gentleman had reached his maximum benefit for acute and subacute rehabilitation. He was then placed a skill nursing facility because there were issues in his care which required the services of a registered nurse (RN). On his admission, he was able to feed himself, propel his wheelchair using the unaffected lower extremity. He was also able to attend to his oral hygiene unassisted. He was in fact someone who did not require total care; this status required less care time to function, and his caregiver was able to devote more time to patients with greater needs. Within a period of twelve months, things seemed to have changed. A person who was functional and independent in several ADL activities had become virtually dependent for all of these activities, including his limited mobility in wheelchair and ability for self-feeding. Advocates for this patient were concerned and sought reason for such precipitous deterioration in his functions. My best response to a complex question was "Disuse. You lose what you don't use." Although the answer is as simple as the expression, it seemed difficult to prevent in many SNFs. It should be appreciated that some of the problems encountered are clearly outside the purview of the local facility and reflect policies dictated at higher levels of management.

My determined effort for an explanation and, therefore, a solution for the deterioration of function of in this patient led me to a retrospective analysis of events. Here is a patient who was able to feed himself but required time to accomplish this goal. It appears that because of time constraint, the caregivers assigned to him decided to do good by helping him along. This was the beginning of a regrettable ending; they reduced his feeding time considerably by feeding him, giving themselves more time to attend the needs of others or fulfilling other functions. On several occasions, he refused to be fed. Apparently, being fed was a humbling experience for him. The act of eating should be a pleasurable one; no one enjoys food being rammed into their mouths to hasten the process when the subject may prefer to be engaged in a civil conversation as he had been accustomed to do. My question would be: Why should it matter if one took forty-five minutes to enjoy his lunch or supper in a skilled nursing facility? This gentleman had a stroke which affected the left extremities but was able to use the right hand. After months of this benevolent care, the patient began to show signs of weakness and restrictions in the right hand and difficulty in his grasp and pinch. Instead of providing a built-up handle to augment his grasp and introduce self-feeding, these deficits were used as an excuse to justify assisted feeding of the client. It was being done and sanctioned by supervisors primarily for the convenience of the staff but to the detriment of the patient. Later, there were restrictions in the right shoulder. It is important to note that the changes in the right hand were taking place without any corresponding extension of the neurological changes noted on his initial examination (CTS); this was confirmed by several subsequent brain scans. Weakness developed in the right hand had more to do with his disuse.

All during this period, there was no structural program to engage the unaffected extremities. To the credit of the facility, there were bingo games, group singing, and storytelling—all sedentary. As weakness progressed in the right hand, there was more difficulty brushing his teeth because he had also lost considerable range in the right shoulder. Eventually, self-feeding and self-oral care were functions of the past; he had become dependent for virtually all ADL functions with little hope of regaining them. It is more achievable to alter the declining process of weakness by physical modalities than to restore strength and functions which were lost by neglect and disuse over time. It would have been easier to delay or abort the rapid deterioration in function of this patient if the caregiver or supervisor had the savvy to deal with the problem. It was easier to feed the client and "get over it." Younger workers tend to show this haste. Some lack the skill and seemed unprepared, although they were willing to learn and were respectful.

One may argue that the deterioration we see in stroke patients and those confined to wheelchairs is the inevitable declining course. It may also be argued that there may also be a declining course in the patient with cardiomyopathy, yet the latter is treated, but the former (stroke) is not. I have taken the opposing view that the course in both scenarios may be altered and requires parallel attention. The concept of "watchful waiting" in these cases have no place in the skilled nursing facilities. Waiting for what? Deterioration! These are our friends and neighbors, many with aspiration and hope; their defaults are the inability to walk and unable to function independently. I have taken on the advocacy of stroke victims and those in SNFs who are sometimes seen motionless, slumped in their wheelchairs, sitting in the full view of the nursing station. I believe their well-being would be addressed if their motor deficits are addressed after the covered period for Medicare/Medicaid expires. The term maximum benefit has become a cliché to imply that payment under Medicare and Medicaid had come to an end, and "you're now on your own." For those with financial means who are able to pay for the cost of ongoing therapy, even limited therapy, will maintain a level of independent function for some time. Those unable to receive these limited services will continue their decline, sometimes painfully.

As more wheel-chaired applicants are admitted to SNFs, programs must be conceptualized to challenge the residual functions of these clients. To begin this process, facilities must acquire the personnel who have the skill and the vision to work with the physically challenged. The staff will then develop and coordinate activities with physical therapy and occupational therapy so that there is notable carry-over on the wards that which is gained during therapy. There are programs and activities which are specifically designed for this group of residents. These activities are geared toward the trunk and upper extremities. Alternatively, a physiatrist, physical therapist, or occupational therapist, experienced with stroke/wheelchair patients, may be consulted to assist in developing ongoing programs. The physiatrist may also be able to set limits based on the medical history of participants.

The most frequently neglected modalities for wheel-chaired patients in SNFs are positioning and application or reapplication of splints and braces. Poor positioning of clients/residents seems to be an endemic problem and is allowed to be perpetuated at all levels of care. Application of braces and other forms of support are modalities which could be addressed by a coordinator. A poorly applied brace could result in irreversible problems for the clients/patients and a legal nightmare for the administration.

An important personnel in the skilled nursing facility is the rehabilitation coordinator; this would be a person with some rehabilitation orientation who would work with both the nursing and physical rehabilitation team. This member will address the many problems which relate to mobility of all residents in the SNFs, especially those confined to wheelchairs. Mobility, including positioning, is among the most common omissions I have encountered in SNFs. When physical therapy/occupational therapy programs are terminated, and with the expiration of Medicare coverage, resident returns to their room and that is the end of their structured physical activities; this does not include the social programs (music, singing, movies, bingo, etc.). To witness those confined to wheelchairs often sitting in front of the nursing station, one would note that there is very little active movements occurring. Apart from the movements of transfer from bed to chair, there is little one observes which could be described as body movements; patients remain almost fixed in the position they were placed by caregivers/aides. For those who receive care in their homes, my preference has been the rocking chair. The clients are often able to rock back and forth with both feet planted on the floor. This simple action is of immense benefit to muscle contractions in the extremities; it also increases circulation and the function of the heart, cardiac output. The coordinator may also be able to implement some form of recreational therapy and activities which involve body movements. It has to be remembered that this form of exercise may be the only exercise feasible for these residents.

The Aphasic Residents: The approach by many caregivers to clients branded as aphasic needs review. The assumption that aphasic patients lack understanding is a serious misconception. There are levels of aphasia so that although a client may have difficulties with fluent expression of his/her thoughts, he/she may have no difficulties in processing or understanding your questions or your commands; with this thought in mind, caregivers should always explain to their clients whatever actions or procedures they intend to pursue. This is also an act of courtesy and respect. Perhaps just as important, you should never communicate in "baby talk" to any of your charges; they may have far more advanced language comprehension than you may have acquired in your lifetime. One patient with moderately severe expressive aphasia wrote, "Why does the aide talk to me like that? I am not a baby." This was a patient who had suffered a TIA (transient ischemic attack) and fully recovered within six weeks.

I share these incidents and occurrences with the hope that they serve some useful purpose for caregivers. Per diem and part-time workers in SNFs are likely to lack many of the basic skills for their job description. Staff training should be an ongoing exercise at skilled nursing facilities (SNF) so that those who may have escaped some of the basics would have an opportunity to receive them. Another justification for this exercise, the turnover of staff is high, and rules and procedures vary from institution to institution. Per diem and part-time workers form an important contingent of workers at SNFs; they are more likely to lack many of the basic skills required of caregivers. Some employers pressed to cover an unexpected opening and have little time or the inclination to find experienced interim workers may be forced to hire workers without the minimum experience required for the task. Institutions which have large numbers of part-time and per diem workers are more likely to offer a lower standard of care than those with regular full-time staff. Absenteeism at these institutions also became a chronic problem, and the cycle of declining standard is perpetuated.

Institutions in remote locations from metropolitan areas find it necessary to offer overtime to its staff at an unprecedented rate. This option may benefit workers whose weekly wages are enhanced; it may also benefit the institution by providing an accessible pool of trained workers. The down side when this practice is abused, the clients/patients suffer from neglect. In a very active workplace, I was able to recognize all those who had worked a double shift without making inquiry. Some walked as though they were heading for the emergency room, some seemed half awake. Sixteen hours a day, twice in a given week and expected to be able to function effectively and serve the needs of sick people is beyond any expectation. Yet expediency forces administrators to resort to these hard choices at the expense of quality care. I have to agree that it is better having some coverage than none; this is the dilemma confronted by administrators. They face a no-win situation, and my observations expressed here imply no criticism of local administrators of the large health care facilities. They do their best under difficult situations.

I see a replica of my tenure as an intern decades past; those were the days when a twenty-four-hour shift once a week was a welcomed treat; but when this occurs three times a week as was in practice, the treat became a treatment and despised by all interns and residents. I remember arriving on duty at 7:00 a.m. for briefing and discussions with the chief resident about the patients admitted on the previous day; these discussions were about management plans. We were expected to give our presentations without reading from the patients' charts, and most of us were able to do this. By 7:30 a.m., it was presumed that the interns had their breakfast between 7:00 a.m. and 7:30 a.m. At 8:00 a.m., it was time for ward rounds, lasting from forty-five to ninety minutes, depending on the rotation, the number of interns in the group, and the temperament of the attending. We were always able to judge the nightlife of our attending by his conduct during ward rounds. The rest of the morning was devoted to patients' care, lectures, conferences, and presentations. We were expected to do blood work, initiating or restarting disconnected IVs, even thoracentesis (aspiration of pleural fluid), extraction of toe nails and the like. During the afternoon, we are expected to be in the various clinics and to attend new admissions assigned to us. For those patients arriving at 3:45 p.m., you are responsible for the completion of the admissions process, including your treatment plan before leaving the ward or the hospital. You may also be on call during the night, a twenty-four-hour day or close to one. In the OB/GYN rotation, the usual delivery calls were 2:00 a.m., and my question was always "Why can't these babies come earlier?" Those days are now looked upon as "the days of yore," even though I was never a sage nor did I wear a pigtail.

Affiliated Training: Many facilities offer contracted arrangements with local colleges, whereby their facilities are used for the clinical training and experience of medical and nursing students. I have supported these arrangements as medical director of a physical rehabilitation service. I believe these arrangements offer benefits to the skilled nursing facility and the college, with colleges receiving a larger portion of the benefits. To offset these, colleges may offer a small stipend to the SNFs; the amount varies from institution to institution. Contracts with offshore medical schools may involve large payments, sometimes open for questions. Benefits to the affiliate college are significant because these clinical experiences are in fact an extension of their professional curriculum. The students receive hands-on training using the patients as their subjects. They also have access to other areas of the institution. The institutions may receive a stipend and helping hands in caring for the patients/clients under their charge. However, there is opportunity for abuse of clients by students who have not had sufficient clinical skill to offer the care they are permitted to give. In private institutions, where clients pay large sums for their care, these arrangements may run counter to the wishes of patients and family members who see this an invasion of privacy by unauthorized students.

Administrators and clinical supervisors must ensure that the utmost respect and courtesy be extended to all those whom they have the privilege to serve. Most patients would agree to interventions by students if this is done in a respectful way, with supervisors carefully explaining the teaching objectives of the institution and the benefits to all parties. Such respect for patients, private or otherwise, cannot be overemphasized. There are, however, evidence of serious infractions when students are allowed to carry out initial tasks without supervision. It is unacceptable to demonstrate to students on a model then have them perform the task on clients/patients without supervision. Nursing, like medicine, involves a practice, and this must be done first under the watchful eye of the tutor, followed by intermittent checks. I have seen students taking liberty of attending to clients/patients without the courtesy of an introduction or the presence of a supervisor.

Skilled Nursing Facility may welcome the fact that students are carrying out tasks normally designated for their staff, a labor saving exercise for the institution since fewer staff may be required to cover a designated area. This accommodation, however, poses serious consequences for the institutions and may open the door for possible litigations if things go wrong, or perceived to have gone wrong, in care. Unscrupulous advocates for patients may use this as a pretext to institute investigation of trivial infractions in care which do occur during normal course of events.

Invasion of clients'/patients' records by students, from their DOB to their chief complaints and diagnosis, is a fundamental right which must be protected; always remembering that the facility may not have received written consent to share these records with students who browse for information. One student is said to have confronted a senior patient after discovering his DOB and innocently exclaimed, "I didn't know you were that old!" This teenaged student had forgotten that after the age of twenty-nine, no one wants to be reminded that "they are that old," a reality she may discover in time.

Urinary Tract Infection and Decubitus: Occurrences which are frequent in SNFs are UTI and decubitus over the heels; these occurrences generally reflect poor supervision and nursing care. The best treatment for these is to prevent them from occurring. When supervision is lax and care is poor, there is higher incidence of these problems, and the cover-ups and denials come into full play. UTI in the skilled nursing community is usually an ascending infection. The precipitating cause is from fecal contamination. Patients, especially those who do not verbalize their needs, are left with fecal contamination for hours without being cleaned. Regularly scheduled check and toileting of these residents will alter the frequency of UTI at these institutions. I have already emphasized the need for proper positioning and rotation of patients, especially those who may be vulnerable. A well-supervised and well-trained staff will go a long way in reducing these problems.

THE LARGER PICTURE

A dilemma: Many of the problems experienced in the health care system are elusive and transcendent; these problems are easier to expose than to solve. The benefactors of health care largess are also multiple and elusive, but to attempt a solution, these problems have to be identified and analyzed by those who are objective and beholding to no special interest group.

Who are the players? They include the innocent, often naïve, patient who sincerely believes that the services are free, so why not "pop in the doctor's office since I'm in the area?" Free to this group of consumers means they were not required to make payment to the physician for his/her services, to the drug store for the tablets they received, or to the vendor for the knee brace he had fitted. I am told that some even forget to say "thank you." The services rendered at the hospital clinic in providing emergency medical care are taken for granted.

The larger benefactors are the pharmaceutical and insurance giants and their loyal lobbyists and dutiful lawmakers. It is ironic that these benefactors of the health care largess vehemently complain about the cost of care, presumably to satisfy the expectation of their constituents, but lawmakers adamantly refuse to enact reasonable laws to restrict wasteful and expensive contracts with the pharmaceutical and insurance conglomerates. Laws which forbid the government from contracting with drug companies for lower-priced drugs hardly benefit the consumer; this is the quick fix that fixes nothing. Although the consumers share some measure of responsibility, they cannot be held to the same level of culpability as those who conceptualize and effect a system of deception which results in gain for themselves and the pharmaceutical companies. Another group of benefactors are the CEOs who feel the need to cut down on quality patient's care, only to enhance their stock options and bonuses.

Education: A starting point to a solution is to educate the general public/consumer in the mechanics of the system, how it operates the legal entitlement of the consumer and the common abuse of the system. Many of the services provided, such as appliances, medications, home care services, should not be perceived as infinite. Any system, government-operated or otherwise, can only contribute from that which it receives. The notion that what the consumer receives in benefit is free should be dispelled and substituted by one which asserts "nothing in life is free." Whatever is paid into the social services pool is paid by tax payers, not the government. Social service agencies do a disservice when they only emphasize the entitlements of citizens to the point of inviting the unscrupulous consumer to access services that are not needed nor beneficial.

What should also be emphasized are the limited availability of many resources and the obligations and responsibilities of those who benefit from them. Services should not be accessed because they are available but because they are needed; the prescribing physicians are the gatekeepers for many services and share a measure of responsibility. In a previous section of this book, I have written about redundancy in prescribing, which imposes needless cost to the system.

In some institutions, especially those in the upper ratings, there appears to be a reversal of the pyramid; management staff becomes disproportionately heavy relative to the "foot soldiers" who carry the weight of the system. One patient described them as "dark suits coffee drinkers." I have taken the view, in defense of this group, that responsible managers are necessary and indispensable in a well-run institution; they conceptualize and effect plans far beyond the scope of the workers at the bottom of the pyramid; they are often able to predict negative outcomes before they occur at tremendous savings for the institution. The reasonable question remains: "Does a small institution require as many administrators as they often employ?" The larger question for the institutions: "Who do they supervise? Who do they manage when the base of the pyramid has diminished in numbers?"

Misplaced priorities: There is the tendency to skew priorities from livable wages for caregivers and lower staff-patient ratio in preference for physical appearances of institutions. The example of a broken and dilapidated shades in a client's room was brought to my attention. The caregiver was unable to close the slots so that light continuously beamed into the client's room day and night; this added much to the discontent and annoyance of the patient. He endured this annoyance for two weeks before the window was measured for a new shade and several days after before the shade was replaced. A parallel occurrence at the entrance hall or the lobby received the immediate attention of management and the problem remedied within days or less. The reason is clear; there are advocates for the lobby and common hallways whose voices are heard. Advocacy for clients/patients, whose fees largely maintain the institution, including the lobbies and hallways, are seldom as assertive and vocal. It is necessary for family members to assume the active role as advocates for their loved ones, regardless of the innuendos and claims of micromanagement and meddling sputtered by many.

I assure you that these personnel would "micromanage and meddle" in precisely the same manner if the table were turned. I am certain about this because I have been on the other side of the coin. However, I do advise reason, discretion, respect for personnel and the rules and regulations governing the institution. If you have the expertise in any discipline of treatment, you would be well advised to "keep it under your hat" but ask the right questions and make comments which are not threatening; be a good listener, even resorting to effacement. Your expertise will eventually triumph. As a practicing medical specialist, the assumption had been that you knew more than your patient or members of their immediate family; now I have come to realize how wrong and erroneous this assumption may have been.

Noise: Another vexing problem to many patients which appear to elude the attention of supervisors and administrators is the level of noise in institutions. This first came to my attention as a patient in one of the best hospitals in the city of New York. I thought that perhaps I was overly sensitive to noise and, therefore, dismissed the annoyance. When my patient complained about noise in the hospital environment and insisted that I find a bed in another location, away from the nurse's station, I then realized that this was in fact a real problem and not my imagination. She complained about a staff member at one end of the hallway yelling to get the attention of her coworker at the opposite end; the time of night seemed irrelevant. This behavior was troubling, especially in a skilled nursing environment. Many of the senior residents are unable to sleep because of preoccupation with their own medical uncertainties. A location in the vicinity of the nurse's station was at one time the most desirable location. There are more to be learned about those for whom we care which only they and their loved ones can fully grasp. Several patients with whom I have spoken would rather forgo the claim of security for the possibility of a restful night sleep relatively free from the "Time Square" atmosphere. What I have found to be especially troubling, none of the offenders believed that calling a coworker at the other end of the hallway or the conversation in the nurse's station could be so disturbing that patients are unable to sleep at nights. With such perception of the problem, there was certainly a dilemma to be resolved. To lodge a complaint is to invite possible recrimination. Seniors and clients in the SNF, assisted care facility, or the independent care facility are entitled to a quiet and restful environment at all times, especially during the night when most seniors are having difficulties falling asleep.

This author has praise for those small facilities which make a difference. These facilities and management staff must be commended for the care they offer and the commitment of their staff. It is not that they do a perfect job which is humanly difficult, but they do their utmost to achieve perfection; the primary objectives seem to focus on the care they deliver to their clients. What I have found to be universal in the delivery of quality care is always the good grace and humanity of those health care workers who toil day after day under difficult conditions and low wages yet able to stimulate and motivate their clients/patients and provide for their needs.

My inside view was an educational enlightenment I would never have acquired by mere book knowledge. It was filled with surprises, challenges, heroic deeds, but also showed the lack of humanity at its worse. If we accept that these workers are the prime movers in the care of our loved ones, shouldn't we be equally concerned about the extent to which they are respected and compensated for the good work they perform? Workers who are respected and are reasonably compensated for their work are more productive and serve the needs of their clients with more humanity and grace.

Abusive behavior in the health care system is not limited to direct physical abuse perpetrated by some care workers. I have equated abusive behavior with those conditions which impose physical or mental sufferings. Executives whose primary interest is profit-based incentives and compensations may deliberately suspend certain vital services. This action reduces cost of operation, thereby increasing profits for the company. The end results of such abuse are pain, anguish, and suffering for the clients/patients; this kind of abuse is elusive, seldom exposed nor criticized, and has an indelible negative effect on senior citizens.

When compensations and incentives become the primary focus, there is danger of human excess in the hands of the unscrupulous. It is hoped that more of these sinister behavior would be exposed and challenged. This is not to imply that executives should not receive fair compensation for their labor, unlike the average compensation of health care workers, nor that investors should not receive adequate return for their investments. It simply means that quality care should not be brokered in order to enhance the opulence of those at the top tier at the expense of those in greatest need and without reasonable alternatives. Under the prevailing circumstances, I believe we should return to thinking with our hearts, even though it was made to pump blood.

There comes a time when it is fair to say "enough is enough" to the excess in compensations and bonuses, except for the care workers who make minimum wage, often requiring another job to survive. These workers remain on the poverty list and struggle to care for their family. When I related my concern about this inequity to a colleague, he said to me, "Randy! You may be right, but you are thinking with your heart." He then asked, "Do you know the purpose of the heart?" I struggled for an answer. He then replied, "It was made to pump blood, not to think." He may have been correct, but the "inside view" has taught me that life is not always measured in physiological terms; there is a good instinct present in all humans but difficult to explain; the difficulty lies in man's inability to discover and enhance its application; this dimension separates us from the lower animals. Perhaps it would have been better if we pumped some conscience and good will, along with the blood in our system. Our sleep at nights may be more restful, psychiatric appointments for depression may be unnecessary; we may require less antacids to aid digestion of our meals and have fewer bouts of gouty arthritic attacks. Our lives would then find more fulfillment and happiness which were never experienced, even with the abundance we receive at the end of each year.

I have the conviction that no one makes it in this world by himself; even those who loudly proclaim to be "self-made" have at some point been given a helping hand. The politicians hanging on the shoulders of their constituents, still proclaiming that they are "self-made;" is it ingratitude or naïveté? How about the extension of public road to your isolated office complex at no cost to you but which enhanced patients' access to your once inaccessible office? Your patients' flow has tripled as a result. This is the helping hand one is often confounded to admit. Call it what you may, some perceive this as welfare, while the recipient sees it as the responsibility of good government exactly as does the Medicaid recipient.

CONSULTANTS: Role of the consultant: We are fortunate to have consulting staff at most of the health care facilities I visited for this publication. I was privileged to serve as a consultant at three institutions and as chief of service and as director of physical medicine at two. I have become quite familiar with the role of consultants. Traditionally, consultants for the various medical specialties are highly trained, skilled, and experienced practitioners who have practiced their specialties for a number of years and known in their respective medical communities.

How are the services of consultants activated? In recent years, some patients have sought the services of consultants by direct visit to their offices without any referrals by their family physicians. It is possible that some of these patients may have been seen as making a routine office visit without a referral by their local physician.

Traditional visits to, and interventions by a consultant normally required a referral by a family physician or general practitioner. The physician sees the patient, and after he determines that the problem requires intervention of a specialized practitioner, he informs the patient, and then he may make consultation for patient to be evaluated by the consultant. Alternatively, patient makes consultation.

Case for a Consultation: A forty-year-old white female, married with two children, was seen by her family doctor because of onset of pain in the right lower abdomen with vomiting and low-grade fever. After clinical examination, the family doctor found elevation of the white blood cells but yet unable to arrive at a clear diagnosis and, therefore, could not evolve a treatment plan. He has decided that the problem may be a surgical one; he then advised the patient or advocate of his intention and sought a surgical consultation to assist him in the diagnosis and management; this is the traditional way a consultation is requested. The surgeon, with the family physician, makes the definitive diagnosis of acute appendicitis, and the patient is treated surgically by the surgeon. There are situations where these formalities may have to be bypassed in order to save the life of the patient. A well-trusted family doctor may elect to bypass the patient or advocate and make a referral.

It must be remembered that a consultation is only a consultation and does not bind the family or referring physician to comply with the recommendation given by the consultant. It is merely another vehicle to perfect one's medical/surgical management. It is also a useful tool to share responsibility and to provide the best options for your patient. It may also serve as a determent to legal challenges.

Consultants, like any member of the medical team, are not exempt from the respectful and courteous approach to patient's care, which have been long established and practiced. I was discouraged to see a consultant who has betrayed this long-established tradition. I observed one consultant, whom I had agreed to have her evaluate and manage a patient with post-seizure convulsions who required titration of her medications. The patient was poorly responsive to any verbal commands; she was disoriented in time and place; she had also contracted aspiration pneumonia.

The consultant entered the patient's room where patient's spouse and other family member were waiting for her arrival. She completely ignored the waiting family as she entered and proceeded directly to the patient, gently patting her cheek. "Jane! Jane! Raise your arm. Raise your arm!" The patient did show some reaction to pain stimulation, but there was no other response. The consultant lifted the sheet covering the patient's legs and said, "Raise your leg! Raise your leg!" There was no response. The patient had a stroke about eighteen months previous with a residual left hemiparesis. As the consultant was exiting the room, the spouse got up, and only then did the consultant give her name. The spouse attempted to give some briefing of patient's history but was interrupted by consultant who sternly said, "I want to know when last she had the seizure!" She was given the time of seizure, and that ended the contribution of the family members who knew more of the patient's history and events which followed, all of which seemed irrelevant to the distinguished consultant.

I have not seen any consultation examination conducted with such brevity nor have I heard of any history taken in such a haphazard and slipshod manner—no reflex taken, no sensory testing, no definitive motor testing on a patient with a history of a CVA. When it became known that a physician was in the room with the family members, a somewhat more respectful and courteous demeanor ensued, but the damage was already done. It was too little too late, an opinion was already formed. An inside view" had already observed and mentally documented the events; it was found to be unworthy of a professional. It is hoped that such evaluation are never accepted by senior medical students nor interns. The approach and the conduct were tantamount to a form of profiling. Difficulties often arise when a bill is presented for payment from such a consultant. There is an immediate denial by family of having agreed to any consultation or having known that consultant. I have known of cases where insurance payments were challenged by patients and with success, all because of a total lack of fundamental human courtesy and respect for patients or their advocates.

Discussing the conduct of this consultant with another colleague, he suggested that she was one the best within that group and meant no disrespect, that she was trained in a country where mores may have been somewhat different in clinical practice and in approach to family members and patients. I have taken the position that what we impart to others are more important than what we intend or believe and often reflects our thoughts. This consultant was not living in the country she was trained and earns her livelihood in country and an environment where mores also differ. She should have no delusion that her world is the whole world. She must adapt.

Excerpts from "The Solitude of Alexander Selkirk" should not be her adaptation:

> I *am* monarch of all I survey;
> My right there is none to dispute.
> From the center all around to the sea,
> I am lord of the foul and the bruit.

FEES FOR CONSULTATION: I was asked by several interested groups to discuss consultation fees. This is not an area I have sufficiently researched to be able to offer relevant information. Medical fees seem to be fertile ground for disgruntled patients or those "with an axe to grind." I can only share my limited experience and understanding. With regard to fees paid through Medicare or Medicaid, I would suggest that readers contact any Social Security office for reliable information on the subject. We do know that fees vary from specialty to specialty, and this is the way it should be; some specialties require much longer time for training and more in-depth skill than others, also have greater possibilities for liability. Fees also vary from location to location, and the reason given has to do with the cost of operating an office or clinic in different locations; this also reflects the cost of living in different localities. There is the claim that foreign-trained physicians tend to charge less than their U.S. counterparts; this assertion I have not been able to substantiate. It is a commonly held belief that private insurance carriers tend to approve higher fees for consultation than Medicare or Medicaid, but the premium payments may also be higher.

Medicare has in the past established certain guidelines to be eligible for payment under the system. In the first place, the doctor must be registered with the system. Guidelines were based on complexity of the examination, the specialty, the actual time spent in evaluation, and whether the visit was an initial visit or a follow-up visit. Visits must be spaced so that four visits within a month cannot be billed as an initial consultation or office visit unless there is a new development. Medicare/Medicaid has estimated time spent for an initial consultation, and this should exceed forty-five minutes. Examination should cover all the systems, except for a limited consultation, and this should be stated. The examination will include a complete history. It is highly unlikely for a practitioner to complete such examination in fifteen minutes. Medicare will usually pay 80 percent of what it approves for the consultation. The patient or his coinsurers are responsible for the 20 percent. The problem for physicians is the amount Medicare approves for the services rendered. I have found that charges by physicians are always higher than what Medicare will approve. When one consultant charged $600 for a fifteen-minutes follow-up and no physical examination, only one question asked by the consultant, "Any new problems?" Medicare, in its wisdom, approved only $120 and paid $96. The patient was responsible for the remaining $24. With reports of increasing fraudulent claims, Medicare/Medicaid has maintained an iron-fist attitude to payments.

There is a popular belief that it is the doctor's responsibility to bill the insurance carrier for the fees charged. Whenever the physician undertakes to accept payments from an insurance carrier, his contract with that carrier, including Medicare and Medicaid is largely as a courtesy for his patients. It is not an obligation. It also simplifies his method of collecting; a phone call to one insurance carrier may resolve payment problems relating to twelve or more patients covered by the same carrier. The doctor enters into a contract to treat an individual patient, not to collect. It cannot be overemphasized that payment of the physicians' fees is the responsibility of the patient, whether or not he/she has insurance coverage. Submitting your insurance claim by the physician is simply another courtesy extended to you.

The Golden Years

INSIDE VIEW: There is one experience in life which all people share in common: We all become older. No one gets younger, irrespective of our station in life. This thought should move us to be more respectful and humane to one another; it should transcend any desire to be enriched from the suffering and despair of others. This reality poses questions and seeks solutions. It is an inevitable reality, whether you are destitute and homeless or infinitely affluent, having no thoughts or concern about how your medical needs would be met in the event of a medical catastrophe.

The bigger question for many then becomes: "What would be the quality of care during later years when we become dependent?" One senior who lived independently in a senior facility confided that she will not visit the skilled nursing section of that facility.

I asked her: "Why wouldn't you want to visit when someday you may have to reside there?"

She answered: "I really don't want to see how they treat the people there."

My view from inside has convinced me that the ambience of the entrance hall and other physical surroundings, while admirable and appealing, do not necessarily translate into humanity or quality care in the twilight years, and that care is not always related to the physical extravagances of some institutions. The needs at this juncture in life are caregivers with hearts and souls to carry out the difficult task of caring; a caregiver recognizes the thirsty clients who may be unable to verbalize their desire for water, to recognize the pain and the suffering of the speechless who sits in his/her wheelchair or in bed and unable to verbalize their needs; a caregiver to position the client in the chair or bed so that the pinched nerve in the neck is relieved. These caregivers become the heroes and heroines in the eyes of the sick and disabled. My view from inside also convinced me that an advocate who shares the principles of humanity and understands the operation of the system could be invaluable.

Advocates whose interest is estate settlement after your demise may not be the ones best suited to oversee your interest in the twilight years, whether they be family members or others. Greed and the greedy human instinct sometimes dominate the equation at a time when you are unable to think, see, or hear clearly, and your only preoccupation is your comfort; these decisions and actions have to be made when there is clarity of mind. The paradox is most people do not wish to confront such possibilities at that time.

The health care dilemma will prevail as long we have those who are willing and able to plunder the system for their exclusive gains at the expense of the dependent ones. In the absence of proper supervision and humane caregivers who share the principles mentioned, skilled nursing care is then relegated to mere custodial occupancy in spite of promises made to influence family members in sending their loved ones to these facilities.

I have given some attention to this period of life which I see as a time of reflection and to ponder over some of the earlier adventures. I am sure some were memorable and evoked smiles and laughter; others may have been adventures but events we preferred to forget. Whatever the reflections may have unfolded, the golden years should spring a new beginning when we make new acquaintances and enjoy life as it is, in its fullness, its beauty, its majesty, and with little thoughts of tomorrow.

Who is responsible for the care or supervision of mom or dad, for aunt or uncle who must now be cared for at home or in an institution? They are still able to function but require assistance with meals, house cleaning, supervision with personal care. This is one of the most difficult and contentious issues to resolve among loving family members, family who see themselves as being closely knit and looked out for one another. Under these circumstances, it would appear that decision, who takes the helm in the care or supervision of Mother, would be a relatively easy one. Such conclusion ignores the human factor and the selfishness in the human spirit when any anticipated task or burden is apportioned to them. When it is time to put up or shut up, they chose the latter.

Here is a typical example of a family dispute arising from the decision to choose a member to assume the responsibility for their parent. The eldest son, John, suggests that their parent should be cared for at home but prefers his sister to undertake that responsibility; she has a bigger house with more room for Mom to enjoy. He is unable to accommodate Mom because his wife felt that too much of his attention would have to be devoted to Mom.

How does the sister feel about that arrangement? "Oh! I can't do it," the sister said. "I have to give too much of my time and attention to the two children, now twelve and fourteen years old. You know what that means! How about Harry?"

Harry, the youngest, said, "My wife has a young child, and caring for Mom at my home will not work. Why not sell the house and let

Mom go to an assisted or independent care facility? She would be happier there."

It is interesting to note how each family member found the arrangement in the home of another member as the perfect and ideal place for a loved one, their mom, but each member found his/her residence unsuited for accommodating mom for all the right reasons. They see all the advantages in the other siblings taking care of their mother and the disadvantages if he/she assumes care. If there was ever a diagnosis as a "selfish monolithic personality," their reasoning and actions would qualify members for such diagnosis.

Their perception of the ideal place for mom was based entirely upon their convenience and a disrespect and disregard for the other siblings. Their reasons and decisions are "gospel" not to be challenged. This dilemma are occurring in a family which is close-knit, but caring for mom results in vengeful family dispute. The solution is always the demise of the family member when those who have contributed the least in care are the first to appear on the scene to demand their share of the undeserved inheritance; this inevitably ends in judicial litigation in which only the attorneys benefit from these misguided events.

In these heated family disputes, the independent living facility (ILF) or the assisted living facility (ALF) is the institution which comes to the rescue of these embattled warriors, offering more consistent care for mom, pop, or other family members in need of assisted care. In our complex society, there seems to be little room in the homes of family members for the elderly relative in need of assisted or supervised care. This observation was valid in homes where two or three bedrooms are unoccupied and family members gross over $400,000 per annum.

What was often ignored by the contentious siblings, before they became successful, these are the very parents who had toiled and sweat, doing two jobs to maintain that son or daughter at the best colleges or universities of the nation. They had denied themselves that necessary vacation, that new outfit for Easter, and tolerated an automobile so unpredictable that public transportation or the bicycle was sometimes preferred, slow but would get them to work on time. These burdens and sacrifices were considered to be obligations of good parenting and not as investments for which future returns were expected. However, it is often forgotten that the eighteen-year-old college student is an adult, eligible to vote and serve his country in the armed forces. Any assistance he receives from his parents ought to be considered as being "over and beyond the call of duty." Many adults (over eighteen years of age) continue to benefit from the generosity of their parents who continue to pay the cost of their college and University education, these parents have given their all because they saw this as their obligation and good parenting for which there was no reward expected. One may ask what obligation does a parent have for an eighteen-plus-years adult?

It is a disservice when siblings who have benefitted entirely from the toils and sacrifices of parents now quibble about lending a helping hand to those parents who are now in need. Young parents must discharge their responsibilities and obligations for their children and support them in their educational pursuits so that they are given the foundation upon which to build a viable future for themselves and their family. Beyond these obligations, you have a responsibility for your future, your senior years. Experience of others have shown that in the present socioeconomic climate, dependence upon children for the responsibility of "senior care" is unrealistic and a utopia. Families today are confronted with an economic environment in which many families break even in their income and expenditures from month to month with little possibilities for meaningful savings for the future; such savings are beyond reach of many household. Perhaps their only alternative is adequate and secured insurance coverage.

My inside view of the health care system has given me a glimpse of its dimension and operations and has exposed me to some conditions and practices unworthy of commendation. The compassion and care shown by many staff members at the bottom of the pyramid were remarkable. I am cautiously optimistic for the future of the health delivery system. I am cautious in my prediction because of decisions and policies made by the anointed few at the top of the pyramid; their primary concern seems to be their annual bonuses and compensations, investors' returns and dividends. These policies are sometimes executed with little regard for their negative effects on the quality care of patients or the stress imposed on the staff who maintains the system. I am optimistic because of the men and women whom I have described as the base and foundation of the system, sometimes regarded as its weakest link. Although human imperfections are sometimes manifested, I see in this group people with hearts and souls, people who come to work each day, sometimes working in a thankless environment, one which hardly compensates them adequately for the work they perform. These are the people who make a difference in the lives of many seniors confined to assisted care and skilled nursing care facilities or in their homes. A number of those I have interviewed have expressed displeasure for the disrespect and condescending attitudes to which they are subjected; I found this to be interesting because it indicates that these concerns are paramount in the minds of workers and take precedence over the small wages they receive. Employers must be mindful of the often expressed thought: "I am paying you a salary for what you do," or "I am paying you good wages." This is as though there is an entitlement to disrespect and abuse the worker because he/she is being paid. Remember, salary is paid for work performed, and there is no other entitlement attached.

Viewing from within, I have also been able to observe firsthand social interactions which were never envisaged as a physician, "looking at the other side of the coin." The extent of camaraderie between black health care workers and white health care workers had been quite remarkable to the extent that a white worker was adamant in defending her African American colleague about whom I had complained for neglect of a patient. I had not seen such a defensive stance in other integrated work population. I hasten to qualify that this has not been statistically tested, but at a glance, I found it to be quite unique to health caregivers who work at smaller institutions. I have also been able to dismiss the notion that black health care workers take better care of their clients/patients than their white counterpart.

Man's inhumanity to man has always transcended race. Patients I have interviewed have showed no racial preference for their care workers but have shown preference for quality and satisfaction of work done. The notion that black caregivers take better care of their black patients than their white counterpart, I have found to be mythical, having little substance and unworthy of serious thoughts. Implanted cameras in a home have revealed a black health caregiver mercilessly physically abusing her elderly bed-bound black client to an extent that she was arrested and charged for the crime. The question of elder care and care in general of patients are reflections of ones' humanity. I have found no racial monopoly on the question of humane care, although I have no statistical evidence to substantiate my casual but consistent observation on this subject.

To our senior citizens and those who find it necessary to make assisted care or skilled nursing care facilities their homes, I feel assured that, in balance, these institutions will continue to serve our needs, but we must continue to be advocates for others long before we become residents of these facilities.

Do not be dissuaded as excerpts from "The Solitude of Alexander Selkirk" may lead you:

> O Solitude! Where are the charms
> that sages have seen in thy face?
> Better dwell in the midst of alarms
> than reign in this horrible place.
> I am out of humanity's reach;
> I must finish my journey alone;
> Never hear the sweet music of speech—
> I start at the sound of my own . . .

When I spoke to seniors living at one of the better senior residential apartment complexes in New York State, the golden years were looked upon with mixed feeling; these facilities provided contracts for assisted care and skilled nursing care if needed. Those with adequate funds who had foresight were able to contract for care for the rest of their lives. Large deposit of several hundred thousands of dollars had to be made; the amount depended on the size of the units and other specifics of the contract. Some contracts offered guaranteed assisted and skilled nursing in later years at no additional cost; others offered rental only; some contracts offered up to 90 percent refund of your initial deposits but at a higher monthly rental cost. All contracts provided meals and some degree of housekeeping. All contracts provided for the use of available social and recreational facilities. Limited health coverage is provided by a resident registered nurse. Group transportation is also provided for shopping, doctor's visits, and the like. There is no doubt that these facilities make every effort to serve the full needs of their residents. The dilemma is presented by the increasing number of seniors who may qualify for these facilities each year and the paucity of openings available at cost that the average citizen could afford.

Many seniors who were unable to obtain the contracted lower rates because of medical reasons are expected to pay the full per diem rates, ranging from a few hundred dollars to well over $500, over $280,000 per annum; the cost rises faster than the cost of living or the wages of the caregivers who sustain the system by their labor. It is estimated that it will take two people fully employed at above average national income to earn this amount of money per year. I cannot resist the temptation to describe these rates as being outlandish at best and obscene at worst. These charges do not include the cost of prescription drugs costing hundreds of dollars for a month supply of thirty pills/tablets, nor do they include the cost of your doctor's visits and fees. Laboratory and x-ray fees are separate entities. I have earlier alluded to the large-scale profits made by drug manufacturers for prescription drugs and over-the-counter (OTC) drugs.

To add fire to fury, several of the doctors contacted were unable to accept new patients. These and other events leave me with the feeling of pessimism for the future of the delivery of health care in the United States. I feel certain that relatively few of the next generation would afford the cost of senior residential care at its current rate of escalation, unless the pendulum begins to swing in the opposite direction, having reached its maximum propulsion.

My optimism is buoyed by daily contact with seniors at various facilities; some seniors get around independently with walker, some with cane, some with motorized scooters; others, though impaired, have tried to maintain a military posture; heads up, chests out, as if preparing to give or receive the "royal salute." There was little slouching to be observed in these seniors and virtually no complaints or mention of disabilities. One resident who seemed to be struggling with her specially adapted rolling walker with meal safely placed in an attached basket reminded me that she was slow reaching her apartment, but she did not consider herself disabled. That was the most remarkable revelation I have heard in my years of practice in physical medicine and rehabilitation and gave me much food for thought. Her thoughts were astounding. "How could I be disabled when I live alone? I get in and out of bed unassisted. I attend to my personal hygiene. I read the newspaper and engage in social activities of my choosing. And I am mobile with the special walker. Have you ever seen a disabled car?" I was asked. "It never moves" was her answer. It was a learning experience. This senior had given me new thoughts about my entire concept of disability as I reflected on the status of a disabled automobile. Her reasoned perception of herself was extraordinary. She was slow in getting around with her walker, but who cares? She was not going to a job; she had already put in her time and had secured her future. She was in fact very much unlike the disabled automobile which the driver could not get started, though it had a tank filled with premium gasoline.

Another startling and inspirational experience: I was sitting in a lobby reading newspaper but mainly observing residents come and go at this beautiful and well-appointed senior residential complex. I have always gotten a better picture of certain disabilities when my patients are unaware of being examined. As I sat there, a senior resident in her eighties caught my attention because of her rather unusual and interesting gait. She navigated slowly with a hiking and shuffling gait, but I was more impressed by the fact that she had no assistive devices. As she seemed to struggle for the door I was perplexed that no one was accompanying her, and a gentleman sitting by the door made no attempt to assist. She managed to exit as the automatic doors opened and an ambulance pulled up near the curb, but the driver remained in his seat and never came to her rescue. I murmured, "Why doesn't he get out and assist the lady?" Then things began to unfold. The senior, instead of going to the ambulance turned right, struggled through several steps and proceeded to a brand new red automobile, opened the door, and sped away, leaving the physiatrist gaping and bewildered. These are the seniors by whom I was inspired.

Seniors at one facility see themselves as people living their lives and going about their routine like any other individual. They do the things they wished and able to do. They may perform their tasks slower and take longer to complete them, but they no longer work for Macy's or IBM and no longer active in their professions. They have all the time to do nothing if they so choose, so what's the hurry? The golden years are intended to do just what they do, never be preoccupied about conditions they cannot change but to change those which they are able to change and keep on inspiring others. Perhaps one of the greatest lessons learned, they never complained of being disabled while the tank still has gasoline to burn and the car is moving.

Senior citizens are among the fastest-growing groups eligible for SNC; they outnumber those with disabling injuries or impairment due to other causes. There is a concern among seniors living independently, about the kind of care they may receive in a skilled nursing facility when or if they require that level of care in the future; these concerns are not inappropriate. Many seniors will not visit a skilled nursing facility, explaining that they would rather not see the kind of environment and care which may be their destiny in years ahead; these are seniors currently enjoying their golden years. To expose them to any adverse possibilities would rob them of the golden years they currently enjoy with little thoughts of tomorrow.

In response to these concerns, I have had discussions with administrators. I was surprised that some adamantly contend that the apprehension of seniors to visit a skilled nursing facility has nothing to do with care or the negative and depressing environment at some SNFs; they assert that the resistance of seniors to visit a skilled nursing facility more to do with the "fear of heir finality." I believe such expressions by administrators are baseless and their own defense of the status quo. The implication clearly suggests the care given and the depressing environment at some SNFs have little or no impact on the decision of seniors to avoid visiting these facilities. Such thinking relieves administrators of any responsibility or reason to improve the living environment or the standard of care they offer.

It may be that some seniors are concerned about their "finality," but my view from inside has not supported this cynical views expressed by supervisors, having interviewed a number of senior residents at various independent living facilities. This is not the kind of rhetoric responsible supervisors should be disseminating in any SNF. Seniors show reasoned apprehension for what some seniors described as subhuman living conditions and care, indifference and on occasion, abusive caregivers and supervisors callous in their remarks. Other concerns are odorous bath and toilet areas, no stimulating programs for those capable of participating, patients left all day without being cleaned or changed, and persistent UTI; residents are left in positions which only hasten their crippling deformities and disabilities.

Meals left until cold before being served to residents who are unable to feed themselves is often a problem. The usual excuse is to say "the resident refused to eat." These are many of the valid fears and apprehensions of seniors who refuse to visit skilled nursing facilities. I would assure supervisors and administrators that these ills far exceeded any conjecture of "finality" in the refusal of many seniors to visiting skilled nursing facilities. There is no place for the knee-jerk denial. The sooner these problems are accepted for what they are, the better it would be for the residents who must endure them. The concerns are about the care seniors will receive at a time in their lives when they are dependent upon others for the very basic needs to sustain themselves. The preoccupation about "finality" is more the thinking of a few who are willing to use this as a pretext to avoid the responsibility for enhancing the environment and to maximize the care provided at all levels.

Statements such as "Some seniors want the stars" are inappropriate, regardless of the intent. If I were to respond for these seniors, I would add, "If you pay $180,000 annually for care, perhaps caviar for dinner should be added to the stars." Some administrators express concern about the care they offer seniors and others under their watch. However, they seem to be unaware about specific problems which are of primary concern to the clients/patients in SNF; they are fed by supervisors with sugar-coated information which do not accurately convey the real concerns of residents. I have previously alluded to directors who showed little concern to having one or two male aides alone in rooms with doors closed, carrying out personal hygiene care on female clients/residents; these seniors are often helpless to refuse such imposition. Few physicians would risk intervention under similar circumstances. A closed door may not always be for the privacy of the client but to offer cover for slipshod and unorthodox way of doing some things. What privacy is needed to flush a gastric tube if it is being done correctly and undue air is not being pumped into the patient's stomach to hasten the procedure? What privacy is needed to turn a client in bed if he is not being dragged by his arm in the process?

There are supervisors who see no adverse effect on clients/patients slumped in chairs or wheelchairs all morning with arms almost reaching the floor. These are the care or lack of care which frightens seniors, not their "finality." Living conditions in SNFs have to be made more palatable for seniors. Living wages have to be shared with the base of the "pyramid," the caregivers; this will attract workers with interest, skill, and empathy, thus improving the quality of care offered to those in SNFs. There is a potential workforce of individuals with interest in the care of seniors and disabled, but they are not attracted to working at skilled nursing facilities because of the low wages and other conditions of work; those who administer may have little alternative but to hire whoever is capable of getting to work daily on time and hopefully of good character.

Although many of those hired were desperately in need of work, they also expressed resentment when asked to carry out the very tasks they were contracted to perform. My inquiry has led me to believe that much of their resentment has to do with the wages they receive for the work they are contracted to do (their job description). This oxymoron I am unable to explain.

I do recall a police department in a large metropolitan city which was criticized for the poor quality of their policing; there were reports of high crime rates, corruption, cooping, and numerous other infractions. Many recruits were selected by families who were already members of the force; high school graduation was the minimum required of applicants. More importantly, the pay recruits received was such that those with higher qualifications would shy away from applying. There seemed to have been little incentive to attract those with higher academic and social skills. Something dramatic and intriguing happened. The salary and benefits for those applying to be police officers went up appreciably; simultaneously, the entrance requirements were raised, requiring college levels for new applicants. I am told that these changes not only increased the number of applicants, but they also increased the quality of applicants and improved the standard of policing. Perhaps health care facilities for seniors and others may benefit by this transformation of policing and apply these principles to SNFs. Remember! Success is largely measured by outcome.

The Golden Years: Gold, silver, and diamonds are often regarded as precious metals and stones. In biblical references, gold and silver were frequently used in reference to the wealth of individuals: "You missed a golden opportunity," implying the best opportunity for a business or other transaction. Today, public good or evil is influenced not by gold but by the dollars one has accrued. However, the golden years for seniors still offer "golden opportunities" and should be cherished and utilized as the important years of their lives. The golden anniversary of a marriage or of a business establishment is set aside as a time of joy and celebration, a time for reflection of ones' struggles and accomplishments. In some measure, it is the time of life to recapture some of the events and frivolities missed in earlier years. I have observed seniors in their golden years at several independent living facilities traverse the halls, browse in the libraries and the recreational areas; some aided by walking cane, some with special walkers, some with motorized chairs; I was impresses and inspired. To hear these seniors laugh during the course of their engagements in card games and other recreational activities, one would believe these laughter were being evoked from the guttural of teenagers; it reflected the depth and breadth of their enjoyment of the golden years with little thoughts of tomorrow; they conveyed a sense of resilience and fortitude one would wish to inculcate.

THE DILEMMA

The dilemma we face in the delivery of health care are many and convoluted but can be resolved if the causes could be recognized and identified and there is a willingness and resolve to correct the problem.

Some have inquired, "Aren't there anything right in health care?" The answer is yes. There are many things that are right in the delivery of health care, and those who are at the helm ought to be commended. However, the things which are right and working well are not usually the causes of "the health care dilemma," the subject of this book. The root causes of our dilemma, in my view, stem from those entities which are not working well or not working at all. "An inside view" brings into focus those entities which are identified as contributing to the dilemma and where the instinct of denials prevent any possibility of remediation. There are leaks in the system.

The following may be an attempt at remediation:

- Identify the entities which are incongruous to the smooth and orderly operation of the system and become problems.
- Willingness to address and to initiate action which will bring about changes; there are those who have all the resources and support but lack the will to do. They procrastinate and equivocate.
- Ability to address problems in terms of their cost and your priorities; administrators may be encumbered by cost constraints or undue pressure from those above whose primary interest is to maintain the status quo usually for ulterior motives.
- Having the technical human resources to carry out the task and supervisors who are able and willing to train and supervise.

My view from within has allowed me to witness occurrences, many of which are well known through press coverage and other venues. I offer no unequivocal solutions to very difficult and convoluted problems seen as "the health care dilemma." It is apparent that the system as presently structured is unsustainable because of the enormous cost of its operation and some of its policies. This simple truth reminds us that a system cannot give more than it receives and continues to be viable and sustainable.

More money into such system without internal reorganization and auditing will not alter the course of its demise. There has to be a complete reorganization of its fiscal structure its operation and its policies. The influx of new funding is certain to create the characteristic vulture-like propensity. Some executives, already grossly overpaid in salaries and bonuses, will be reaching out for their largess. The pharmaceutical conglomerates and other giant suppliers will follow the lead and grab their share. The insurance magnates will not be left out while the cost to the insured and others escalates. Regrettably, the wages of caregivers and those who produce goods and services remain flat.

To keep shareholders happy with their dividends, executives and their mouthpieces will balk at any attempt to increase the minimum wage of $7.75 per hour. Their solution is to consolidate services and operations, appoint more top executives, fire the workers who sustain the health care pyramid I have described. More millionaires are created at the apex while the base sinks further into poverty and despair. The fort must be held, but why at the expense of the most vulnerable and least compensated of the pyramid, the health care workers? Increased cost in operation of the system hardly ever translates into increased wages for this level of workers. It invariably translates to increased salaries and bonuses for the top few. There must be a way to reduce the excesses at the top, including the suppliers of medicines and equipment, and equitably reward those who sustain the system, the caregivers at the bottom.

The sad realities: One of the richest countries in the world is said to spend more per capita on health care than any other developed country, having the best care institutions and health care personnel but fails to deliver care to its people in a comparable manner. The system must prove that it is capable of spending funds made available, within the constraints of affordability if the dilemma is to be resolved.

Cost at all levels must be brought under control, but like the contentious family who refused to accept responsibility for the care of mom, no contributor to the health care dilemma is willing to accept any measure of responsibility and come forward with viable propositions to resolve the problem. Some professionals, physicians and others, who expressed willingness to take some responsibility, fault some users of the system who will always be dissatisfied, demanding, and unreasonable. One practitioner, after billing one of his patients for

$125 for an initial consultation, was challenged by the patient about the fees charged. She told him; "few people make $50 an hour." She may have been correct, but what she did not factor into these nominal charges were payment for an assistant and receptionist/secretary, payment for rental of the office where she was examined, insurance payments for staff. Only after these mandatory payments are made could the practitioner receive his salary from which his own insurance premiums and licenses fees have to be paid. The patient concluded that the "problem with health care was one of dollars and cents."

What this well-meaning citizen failed to realize, that we do live in a capitalist society which she enjoys and this is the way it operates. The greatest incentive is to make money and more money. The system works well but there must be a balance. My greatest concern, however, is that we overreach as the trend now indicates and relegate human values and morality to the back burners and obfuscate our principles. The dollar then controls all of our actions. It is perhaps time for the pendulum to begin its backward journey; the laws of gravity will intervene. When maintaining a senior in a skilled nursing facility as much as $200,000 a year, plus a 6.8 percent tax in some states, a merciless addendum, regardless who makes the payment, we are creating a health care monster for the rich and powerful, which in time may destroy itself. To dramatize this reality means it will take the gross annual income of three average middle-income working families to maintain one single individual in a skilled nursing facility (SNF). This reality boggles the mind and shatters the imagination of many, so the perspicacity of those who would descent has been disabled. I must again ask, "Where are the merciful?"

"All that glitter is not gold," and seniors should be cautioned that entering into a skilled nursing or memory care unit from your contracted independent living status may have some encumbrance. Administrators are said to hinder such transfers, giving preferences to applicants who have no contracted agreement with the facility. It is all about money and poses a dilemma for seniors who had the erroneous impression of an orderly and automatic transfer from their independent status. Charges for SNC may run as high as $600 a day. When scruples are influenced by dollars, even the merciful may forgo the reward of mercy and deny your application, giving preference to applicants who are willing and able to pay these outrageous fees for room and board plus additional state tax when applicable.

No one will deny that health care facilities for seniors have made tremendous strides over the years. Some seniors were able to plan their care in advance of later years. They are now able to contract with health facilities of their choice. Perhaps the greatest advantage, an individual may be able to live in an apartment or a bungalow as long as he/she is able to maintain an independent living status. When this status changes and they require assistance for certain daily living needs, they have the option of scaling down their lifestyle to other living accommodations better suited to their functional needs and within the confines of the same institution. At a later stage, if skilled nursing becomes necessary, a further change in care plan may be made for care within the same institution and at no additional cost to the resident. Advance planning gives peace of mind which abates the frustration and anxiety many encounter at this juncture of their lives. Unfortunately, the initial cash payment to enter these facilities precludes many seniors from taking advantage of these limited facilities. It is reassuring that long-term insurance, especially when initiated earlier in life, may mitigate cost if one becomes disabled.

SETTING THE TONE: Long-Term Facilities/Skilled Nursing Facilities: The high cost of care in these facilities continues to be issue of great concern. As I observed administration at various health care facilities, I note a striking correlation in quality care with the demeanor and dress appearance of caregivers. Almost without exception, the standard and quality of care could be predicted by these entities. It is presumed and with some justification that an administration that tolerates or acquiesces to infractions of certain rules of conduct, demeanor and dress will also tolerate behavior and actions by members of their staff, which may be detrimental to residents under their care. By convention, the institution decides whether or not a dress code should be in place; this requirement is not within the purview of residents nor their family members. To impose a dress code for caregivers raises the question: Who bears responsibility for the cost involved? Employees contend that with the miserly wages they receive, imposition of a dress code would reduce their wages. The cost they contend should be the responsibility of employers. When unions are involved, this issue is settled at the bargaining table. Employers contend that everyone dresses for work, and they simply request that dress for the positions offered (health caregivers) requires certain uniformity in dress. They further contend that police and firemen wear uniform. The extreme example: Sanitation employees also wear uniform. In support of a dress code for health care workers, I have experienced health care workers dressed in "whatever they wished," sometimes with costumes better suited for the sunny beaches of Florida and presenting an impression of chaos and disorder. Some structure is needed in the appearance of health care workers at institutions. These and other issues should be clarified at time of employment, before the worker is hired, that a dress code is mandatory for the position being offered.

The rules are set before the worker is employed. The deportment of employees and supervisors should be exemplary. Some who have studied and analyzed behavior have concluded that the way one dresses often influences behavior. An individual attired in a formal dress suit is less likely to start a street brawl than the same individual in his work clothes as a mechanic or other blue collar workers. Another entity which has influenced quality care is the tone/temperament of supervisors and the staff they supervise. Supervisors and staff members who congregate at nursing stations, some sitting on desks while patients are slumped uncomfortably in their wheelchairs, send a chilling message to visitors and advocates. This is more reminiscent of a barroom environment and should never be encouraged at any time. When one charged with the responsibility of directing/supervising a service is himself hostile and belligerent to staff and advocates for residents, such behavior portends adversely to the quality of care offered at that community. Reports of supervisors chastising family members or staff in the full view of patients go far beyond the expected norm. The larger question: Who supervises the supervisors? These are the very residents and family members whose fees and support sustain these institutions, and nothing should be done to encumber their well-being. As outlandish as these revelations appear they do occur, some of which never gets the attention of administrators. It should always be remembered that the tone set implicitly creates a platform for behavior and conduct. It may also be an index of the care to be anticipated.

EDUCATION/TRAINING: It is now believed that health care at home and at the various institutions is one of the fastest-growing industries in the United States. As the senior population grows and the need for senior care increases, there will be greater demand for senior accommodations. What will not increase proportionately is the number of skilled personnel to care for this growing population. The prospect of correcting this potential imbalance seems uncertain because there is a decline in the number of performing high school graduates who are attracted to this level of health care, the caregivers, and the number of male graduates with interest is even lower for workers interested in senior care.

Cursory observation shows a large number of minority workers, recent immigrants, and those with GED certification make up a large number of the workers engaged in senior care. Those with creditable high school certification and college degrees hold supervisory positions, including most of the registered nurses (RN). This correlation between job class with education/training has raised interesting questions and possibilities for those who would take advantage of the educational opportunities available in various areas of health care. It also points to opportunities which are available and those anticipated for qualified health care personnel. The need for education had been highlighted by the president of the United States and Mrs. Obama who emphasized that "education is the road to the middle class." This slogan applies to education in general.

There is a growing need for qualified caregivers to the extent that institutions are forced into employing some with questionable skills or temperament for the positions available. I have observed that those institutions placed at these disadvantages inevitably offer a lower level of care. This dilemma is exacerbated where there is no in-house training program and a discordant supervisory staff; those unsuited for staff positions are also likely to increase as the pool of trained/qualified applicants diminish.

A helpful tool in resolving the problem is the education coordinator who is knowledgeable in senior care and familiar with the physical and mental problems peculiar to seniors. Such coordinator should be a hands-on personnel with applied knowledge, not merely to sit behind the computer entering information, many of which had not been carried out during course of that day. The need for documentation, as important as it is, has resulted in registered nurses (RN) functioning as ward clerks documenting details. Visitation with patients/residents and on-site observation to ensure that care plans are carried out are events of the past. This dichotomy from nursing has reached a point at some institutions that one can no longer expect information about the status of your patient from the RN in charge. In an efficiently operated institution, there should be time for documentation and time for interaction with patients and staff.

Institutions must take more responsibility for the training of the care workers they employ, if they are to expect quality care for their patient population. Internship and residencies structured for medical graduates have served the profession and hospitals well. There was the realization that four years of medical training, even though this may result in successfully passing the state boards, does not adequately prepare the physician to be engaged in the independent practice of medicine. In addition to residency requirement, some specialties expect additional experience obtained though fellowship programs. This background training for physicians assures a higher quality of trained medical personnel. These physicians in training do receive stipends during their training to offset the cost-of-living expenses. Although caregivers are not being trained as physicians, the principles in training for enhancement of skills have some relevance. Like physicians, care workers require training above that which they receive at the various training centers. Many of those I have observed are in dire need of mentoring. I have seen recently trained workers forcing large volume of air in flushing a gastric feeding tube unaware of its consequences. In one instance, there was a recently trained employee who had been on the job for two weeks, instructing a new comer in applying a bandage; unfortunately, the application was tighter proximally and resulted in a large swelling of the patient's foot, the very problem for which the bandage was being applied. These infractions are often dismissed by supervisors as being trivial, and this acquiescence enforces the wrong climate in care and denotes the quality care offered by such institutions. The willingness to excuse bad habits and practices by some workers is perhaps one of the worst transgressions in senior care; it results in needless pain and suffering to the most vulnerable, our seniors and disabled. These candid observations and comments are not to imply that all care are carried out at this level of performance. There are countless numbers of exemplary workers who work against odds to ensure safety, health, and well-being of their charges. Expression of appreciation for these services are often neglected by clients and their advocates.

JOB/WORK SATISFACTION: Satisfaction derived from caring for seniors is presently very low. Many of the workers I have interviewed were dissatisfied with the work they do. Some remarked, "Well! It's just a job." This view was expresses by most of the younger workers. After a glimpse of their job description, I concluded that the main reason for the dissatisfaction by young people relates to the perception and the reality of the job as just a "mechanical exercise." They are asked to give baths or showers, to dress and convey patients to other areas of care; they assist in feeding and toileting. "There is nothing intellectual, exciting or challenging in any of the things we do." This was the view of several of the young men I interviewed, and it was difficult to offer rebuttal.

How can this work (caregiving) be made more appealing and more challenging to more people, especially in the younger age group? As I commiserate with these young people I sense their frustrations and disappointments. I believe it is a natural desire to experience meaning and purpose in the work we perform, something we can relate to friends. Caregivers must be made to experience and appreciate the important therapeutic aspects of their work. A bath should not be seen merely as a mechanical action requested by a supervisor. The therapeutic value of bathing should be explained: It involves controlled water temperature; the application of an antiseptic agent, the soap; the ranging of the client's extremities. The caregivers in fact, are administering valued therapy. During the act of lifting or transferring, caregivers must be made to experience and appreciate their important function in the protective and therapeutic action of a bed transfer, bed rotation, or bed positioning. These procedures are more than the movement of an object; they constitute a measure of therapeutic exercise being given to their charge; this fact must be made known during these procedures. In the application of oils and ointments, which are often applied by caregivers, there must also be acknowledgment of the therapeutic value of these procedures so that there is meaning to the task they perform.

At present, there is a disconnect in what they do as caregivers and their importance as members of the treatment team. The caregivers also deserve time for case presentation and discussion with their peers. At the end of their tour of duty, they should see themselves as important members of a treatment team. When one performs work that many are reluctant to undertake, a measure of respect goes a long way to soften the impact of a job considered less desirable by many. Administration must do what is necessary within its constraints to enhance the feeling of worth, self-respect, and the important contributions of these workers. To upbraid workers by belligerent supervisors in an audience of patients and other workers not only belittles the workers but it also belittles the supervisors; these practices are not uncommon and have direct influence on care and on the ability of supervisors to supervise. Some caregivers complain that they have no decent place to sit and enjoy their meals like human beings; others complain about the number of patients assigned to one caregiver. At one institution, the ratio was one to twelve; this was given the lowest rating on the quality care assessment table I have devised. I have *had* elements of these complaints at every institution observed for this book.

COST: There is cost increase in the delivery of health care either at home or at an institution; the way the charges are evolved by various institutions poses a dilemma to those who are responsible for payments. **There appears to be a deliberate and concerted attempt to confuse the issue of cost and there are always willing hands to effect this confusion.** The cost incurred by frequent and indiscriminate use of the emergency rooms and doctors' offices has not helped the cause of fiscal restraint. The notion that somehow the services are free must be dispelled. I have previously alluded to excessive prescribing, padded fees for services, and excessive charges for appliances and equipment. Waste and pilfering within the institutions are not uncommon and must be addressed by the respective institutions. Mention is made because many of the charges incurred are billed to the health care system, Medicare and Medicaid. Many of us have read reports about hospital cost published by the state Department of Health. These reports expose cost differential of hospital care at various hospitals and cover identical procedures. Many were shocked to note the discrepancy between actual cost for a procedure and services and the charges which were submitted for payment. At one institution the cost to the hospital was stated as $11,000, but the charges submitted for payment were $51,000, about four times the actual cost. There was no reasonable explanation nor transparency for the charges submitted. To state that the payments for care are covered by insurance carriers is to assert the arrogance of those responsible for redundant charges perpetuated with absolute impunity and with no apparent concern for consequences.

Individual agencies responsible for payments of these charges should also be faulted. Why would any agency pay out millions of dollars without a proper cost assessment and verification of the merits of the claims? This points to weakness in the system which ought to be addressed. Alternatively, the excess in payment should be refunded to the health agencies involved. Anyone reading the reasons and explanations given for the cost/charges submitted by the various institutions and individuals is bewildered. **Explanations vary from: "Charge is never what we charge one patient and its just a number we have in our system;"** Another reported, "Hospital pricing is complicated and based on a set of comprehensive algorithms." These statements are nebulous and offer no meaningful explanation to ordinary readers. To state that insurance pays the cost of these charges is to enforce their justification without offering any valid or plausible explanation for such outrageous discrepancies. Although insurance carriers may have picked up the tabs in some cases, the plight of the uninsured was unresolved, and the discrepancy between cost and charges was left dangling. The explanations offered by these institutions were questionable. Cost escalation is not unique to institutions; other groups and individuals have also contributed to this dilemma in the delivery of health care.

There is yet hope and expectation that health care for more Americans will be a reality. The pace of universal health coverage is painfully slow, but this must be considered in the context of time. Today more people benefit from some form of health care with the advent of Medicare and Medicaid; these health care umbrella were thought to be socialistic and were forcefully resisted by some of those who are today thankful beneficiaries of the programs.

How can we improve on the quality of care delivered to patients? This may be achieved by improving and increasing the quality of training for those entering the system. Proper training for those who support the system, "the pyramid," has apparently regressed, and there appears be a lack of interest by younger people. This disinterest relates to the low pay scale offered to this group of workers, consequently a lower estimation of the job as a vocation. One young care worker asked, "How can I support a family on $8 an hour?" I believe that training, better wages, and more respect for workers will promote a sense of job pride and will alter this declining trend.

Quality care for seniors and others will continue to improve with improvement in the quality of training and improved wages. When systems are operated primarily for the benefit of CEOs and directors who operate them, rather than the people they serve, there will be fractures in the system. It should, however, not be forgotten that investors deserve fair returns for their investments if the system is to function for the benefit of all: the employees, the investors, and the people they serve.

The escalation of cost must be vigorously pursued, whether those responsible are influential institutions, pharmaceutical conglomerates, insurance giants, or the ordinary public at large; these should be brought to justice, to establish guilt or innocence.

A care-free environment must be established so that wherever one lives, the golden years should be one of reflections, satisfaction, and enjoyment.

INDEX

A

absurdity, 72, 104, 143, 146, 150
abusive behavior, 40, 189
access to water, 170
accommodations, 98-100, 102, 106, 120, 213, 215
acetylsalacetic acid (Aspirin), 147
activities, 46, 68, 79, 87-89, 95-96, 100, 102, 109-10, 117, 123, 126, 128, 170-71, 173, 176-77, 179-80, 204, 208
activities of daily living, 95, 123, 126, 173
actuary, 129
adduction, 75, 77
administrators, 10, 22, 29, 34, 38, 43, 54, 64, 77, 79, 83, 87, 92, 112, 120-21, 137, 149, 169, 173, 176, 182-83, 187-88, 205-6, 210, 212, 215
advance planning, 213
advisors, 130
advocates, 36, 53-54, 68, 82, 97, 99, 104, 114, 121, 150, 162-70, 177, 184, 187-88, 191-93, 197, 202, 214
Affiliated Training, 183

Affordable Care Act, 37, 67, 112, 142
African Americans, 36, 173, 201
air mattress, 53, 169
Alice (my girl), 30-31
Alzheimer, 30, 124
ambulance, 17, 204
ambulation exercise, 72
American-born, 36-37, 45, 158
American citizens, 159
American consumers, 147
American counterparts, 38
American household, 38
American Medical Association, 70
Americans, 21, 23, 36, 45, 57, 94, 102-3, 105, 130, 142-44, 149, 173, 220
American workers, 38, 157
antibiotics, 112, 140
apartheid, 14
aphasia, 176, 180-81
applicants, 34, 36, 38, 40, 52, 55, 57, 66-67, 91, 96, 98, 107, 124-25, 173, 175, 179, 207-8, 212-13, 215
Archives of Physical Medicine and Rehabilitation, 111
Archives of Physical Medicine and Rehabilitation, 111
army sergeant, 47

221

X

Y

CPSIA information can be obtained at www.ICGtesting.com
Printed in the USA
BVOW04*2121141014

370655BV00002B/3/P